Moving and Handling Patients
at a Glance

3·30·16

WITHDRAWN

Moving and Handling Patients

at a Glance

Hamish MacGregor
Docklands Training Consultants Ltd
14 Roffey Street
London, UK
www.docklandstraining.com

Series editor: Ian Peate

WILEY Blackwell

This edition first published 2016 © 2016 by John Wiley & Sons Ltd.

Registered office:	John Wiley & Sons, Ltd, The Atrium, Southern Gate, Chichester, West Sussex, PO19 8SQ, UK
Editorial offices:	9600 Garsington Road, Oxford, OX4 2DQ, UK
	The Atrium, Southern Gate, Chichester,
	West Sussex, PO19 8SQ, UK
	350 Main Street, Malden, MA 02148-5020, USA

For details of our global editorial offices, for customer services and for information about how to apply for permission to reuse the copyright material in this book please see our website at www.wiley.com/wiley-blackwell

The right of the authors to be identified as the authors of this work has been asserted in accordance with the UK Copyright, Designs and Patents Act 1988.

Library of Congress Cataloging-in-Publication Data

MacGregor, Hamish, author.
 Moving and handling patients at a glance / Hamish MacGregor.
     p. ; cm. – (At a glance)
 Includes index.
 Summary: "Moving and Handling Patients at a Glance provides an accessible introduction to the key theoretical underpinnings of moving and handling, including the legal aspects, biomechanics, risk assessment and safe principles of handling"--Provided by publisher.
 ISBN 978-1-118-85343-6 (paperback)
 I. Title. II. Series: At a glance series (Oxford, England).
 [DNLM: 1. Moving and Lifting Patients–methods. 2. Moving and Lifting Patients–nursing. WY 100.2]
 RM700
 615.8'2–dc23
                                                                                              2015033803

A catalogue record for this book is available from the British Library.

Wiley also publishes its books in a variety of electronic formats. Some content that appears in print may not be available in electronic books.

Cover image: Photograph courtesy of Hamish MacGregor

Set in 9.5/11.5pt Minion Pro by Aptara, India
Printed and bound in Singapore by Markono Print Media Pte Ltd

1   2016

Contents

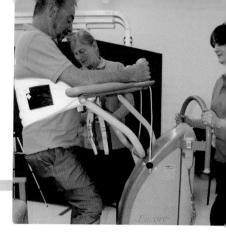

Preface

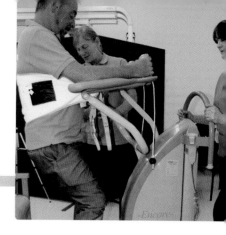

The purpose of this book is to act as a reminder of how some moving and handling techniques are carried out. It is not a substitute for moving and handling training where you have had an opportunity to discuss, observe, practise and ask questions related to moving and handling. There may be some techniques that may differ in their execution from ones you have received during training or carried out in practice. This does not necessarily mean that one is right and the other is wrong, but there are often some minor differences in the way that techniques are carried out. As long as the safe principles of handling can be applied and a rigorous risk assessment has been carried out in the case of an individual patient, then the technique should be acceptable.

Throughout the book I have used the term handler. The reason for this is to use a neutral descriptive term that covers carer, nurse, therapist or anyone who is involved in the moving and handling of people.

I have also used the term patient. This term is to cover not only patient but client, service user, resident or anyone requiring assistance to be moved and handled.

The book is organised primarily as a practical textbook with the theory section at the beginning kept to a minimum. The reason for this is that there are other publications out there that deal with the theory of moving and handling extensively. I am often asked in training, 'Do you have any pictures of that?' hence the emphasis for this book. The techniques described are broken down into their component parts; therefore you may have to read a few chapters to get all the information on moving a patient in a particular situation. This is deliberate and is to maximise the amount of information given in as succinct a way as possible.

To use this book effectively, always read the text first as you are following the pictures on the opposite page. Looking at the pictures and their captions alone will not give you sufficient information.

The primary audience for this book is student nurses, but students of occupational therapy and physiotherapy could also find the book useful. The book may also be a good reference guide for anyone working in health and social care.

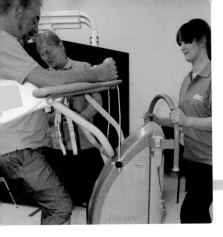

Acknowledgments

I would like to thank Keith Parkinson, my partner and co-director of Docklands Training Consultants Ltd, for his support in compiling this book and assisting greatly in the taking of hundreds of photographs. I would also like to thank Penny Clayden, Lyn Maddams, Glynis Watson and Teresa Yiannaco, freelance trainers with the company for their input in the development of this book — without this, the book would not have come to fruition. Finally I would like the thank Lewisham and Greenwich NHS Trust for allowing us to use their training rooms to take the photographs.

Hamish MacGregor

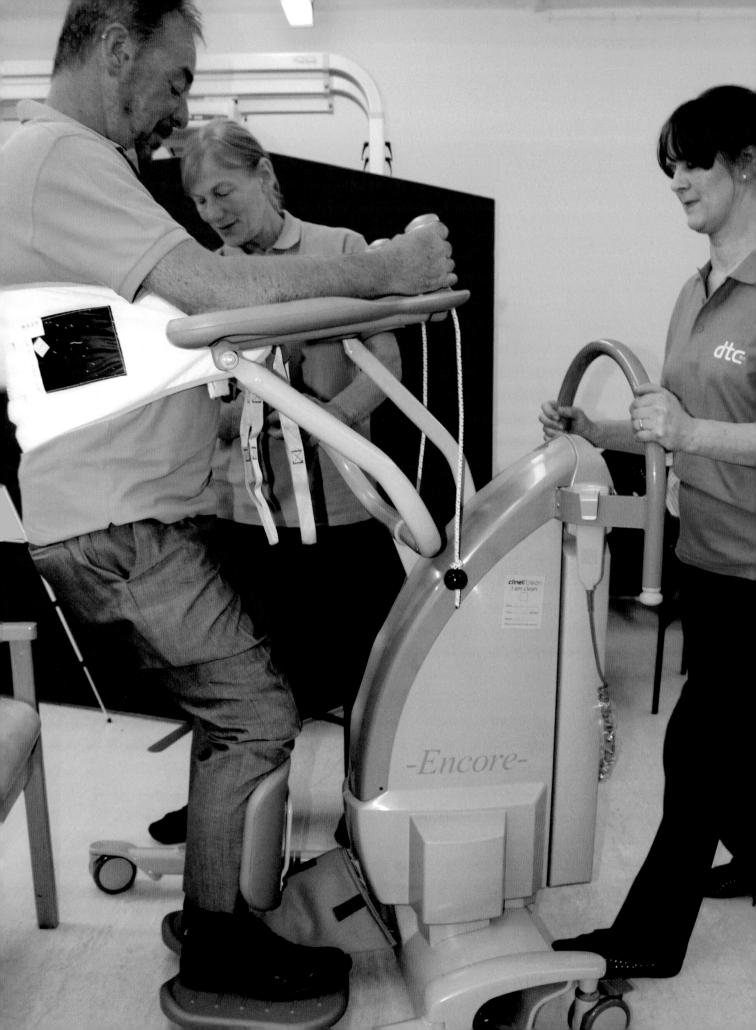

Theory

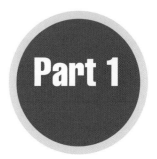

Part 1

Chapters

1 Legislation: I

Figure 1.1 The Health and Safety at Work Act 1974 (HSWA)

Requires the employer to:

- Provide safe equipment and a safe system of work.

- Provide safety in connection with the use, storage and transport of loads (including people) and substances hazardous to health.

- Provide information, instruction, training and supervision.

- Maintain a safe working environment.

- Provide a written health and safety policy statement.

Requires the employee to:

- Take reasonable care of their own health and safety and others which may be affected by their acts or omissions.

- Not damage or disable equipment.

- Be willing to receive training.

Figure 1.2 The Management of Health and Safety at Work Regulations 1999 (MHSWR)

- Risk assessments are required to be carried out by a competent person. A competent person can be defined as a person having the necessary ability, knowledge, or skill to do something successfully.

- In order to carry out the risk assessments hazardous activities in the workplace need to be identified.

- **Hazard** is defined as something with the potential to cause harm.

- **Risk** is defined as the chance or likelihood that harm will occur.

- Risk needs to be reduced to: 'so far as is reasonably practicable'.

Figure 1.3 Manual Handling Operations Regulations 1992 as amended in 2002 (MHOR)

The employer has a duty to:

- Avoid manual handling tasks so far as is reasonably practicable.

- Assess all handling tasks where there is a perceived risk.

- Reduce the risk as far as is reasonably practicable.

- Review all assessments as changes take place and/or at regular scheduled intervals.

The employee has a duty to:

- Follow appropriate systems provided for the handling of loads by the employer.

- Report accidents and *near miss events*.

This chapter covers three areas of legislation that relate to moving and handling. Chapter 2 will deal with four other areas. This is not a complete list but examples of the major pieces of legislation affecting moving and handling practice.

The Health and Safety at Work Act 1974 (HSWA)

This act and its regulations impose a duty of care on every employer to 'ensure as far as is reasonably practicable, the health, safety and welfare at work of all employees'. It not only puts duties on the employer but the employees too. A résumé of the act is given in Figure 1.1.

The HSWA is a broad piece of legislation and could be described as an umbrella that covers a raft of other legislation that is more specific in its nature to moving and handling. The key areas are two-fold: first, the provision of equipment and a safe system of work to accompany this; second, the provision of information, instruction, training and supervision. The key to good moving and handling practice is not only good training. This should provide the handler with the skills to handle patients safely without injuring the patient or themselves. As important is that the handler has sufficient competent supervision in the workplace to ensure that good practice is maintained.

In addition the employees have to be willing to receive training. This puts responsibilities on the handler to ensure that they attend moving and handling training if it has been provided and they have been given the time to attend. The specifics of training are not defined, but terms such as 'understandable' and 'suitable and sufficient' are often used. This allows for a degree of creativity in delivering training so that on the job training can be as effective, if not more, than classroom-based training. The important thing is that any training carried out must be documented as to its content, date of delivery and where, with the handler and the trainer signing a document confirming this. If this does not happen then in the case of injury to staff or patient it is not possible to prove what training has taken place.

For more information on the HASWA see link below:
www.hse.gov.uk/legislation/hswa.htm

The Management of Health and Safety at Work Regulations 1999 (MHSWR)

These regulations set out broad duties for improving health and safety, and introduce the requirements for risk assessment and health and safety.

The MHSWR require employers to carry out risk assessments on tasks considered to be hazardous in the workplace and reduce risks to a reasonably practicable level. These risk assessments must be carried out by a competent person.

A résumé of the main terms of the regulations is given in Figure 1.2. The term reasonably practicable is used in the regulations and there is a definition of this term below.

Reasonably practicable means that which is, or was at a particular time, reasonably able to be done to ensure health and safety, taking into account and weighing up all relevant matters including:

a The likelihood of the hazard or the risk concerned occurring.

b The degree of harm that might result from the hazard or the risk.

c What the person concerned knows, or ought reasonably to know, about the hazard or risk, and ways of eliminating or minimising the risk.

d The availability and suitability of ways to eliminate or minimise the risk.

e Assessing if the cost of eliminating or reducing the risk is grossly disproportionate to the actual risk.

The general terms of the MHSWR can be easily applied to moving and handling activities, but the Manual Handling Operations Regulations 1992 as amended in 2002 (MHOR) are regulations that apply directly to the area.

Manual Handling Operations Regulations 1992 as amended 2002 (MHOR)

These regulations again define the responsibilities of employers and employees.

The MHOR also gives us a definition of manual handling:

• Any transporting or supporting of a load (including the lifting, putting down, pushing, pulling, carrying or moving thereof) by hand or bodily force.

The definition of a load by the Health and Safety Executive (HSE) defines it as 'a discrete moveable object. This includes, for example, a human patient receiving medical attention…'

A résumé of the MHOR is given in Figure 1.3.

The interpretation of the MHOR directly affects all moving and handling practice. Avoiding patient handling is usually about maximising patient independence and constitutes the first key safe principle of moving and handling (see Chapter 5, Key safe principles of moving and handling). Assessing risk is key to all good patient handling and forms a cornerstone of good practice and the MHOR gives us a framework to carry this out (see Chapter 7, Risk assessment). The understanding of the risk assessment process allows the handler not only to 'follow appropriate systems provided for the handling of loads by the employer' but give them the tools to change the way the patient is moved as the patient condition changes.

For more information on the MHOR see link below:
www.hse.gov.uk/pubns/books/l23.htm

Legislation: II

Figure 2.1 Lifting Operation and Lifting Equipment Regulations 1998 (LOLER)

- Lifting equipment should have adequate strength and stability for its proposed use.
- Risk from positioning and installing lifting equipment be minimised as far as is reasonably possible.
- Equipment has to be marked indicating its safe working load.
- Equipment which lifts people to be examined by a competent person at six monthly intervals.

Figure 2.2 Provision and Use of Work Equipment Regulations 1998 (PUWER)

- Ensure work equipment is used for operations for which it is suitable.
- Is maintained efficiently and a maintenance log is kept up to date.

Figure 2.3 Reporting of Injuries, Diseases and Dangerous Occurrences Regulations 2013 (RIDDOR)

What are 'reportable' injuries?

The following injuries are reportable under RIDDOR when they result from a work-related accident:

- The death of any person (Regulation 6).
- Specified injuries to workers (Regulation 4).
- Injuries to workers which result in their incapacitation for more than 7 days (Regulation 4).
- Injuries to non-workers which result in them being taken directly to hospital for treatment, or specified injuries to non-workers which occur on hospital premises (Regulation 5).

Figure 2.4 Two areas of The Human Rights Act 1998

ARTICLE 3: PROHIBITION OF TORTURE

- You have the absolute right not to be tortured or subjected to treatment or punishment which is inhuman or degrading.

ARTICLE 8: RIGHT TO RESPECT FOR HOME, PRIVATE AND FAMILY LIFE

- A person has the right to respect for their private and family life, their home and their correspondence.

Moving and Handling Patients at a Glance. First Edition. Hamish MacGregor. © 2016 John Wiley & Sons, Ltd. Published 2016 by John Wiley & Sons, Ltd.

Lifting Operation and Lifting Equipment Regulations 1998 (LOLER)

This regulation is aimed at ensuring that all lifting operations are properly planned, lifting equipment is used in a safe manner and that, where necessary, it is thoroughly examined by a competent person.

To decide whether LOLER applies it is necessary to answer two questions – *is it work equipment* and, if so, *is it lifting equipment*? The fact that equipment is designed to lift or lower a load does not automatically mean that LOLER applies. The equipment needs to be defined as 'work equipment' which is defined under the Provision and Use of Work Equipment Regulations 1998 (PUWER) (see below).

The definition of 'lifting equipment' is where the equipment lifts and lowers as its *principal* function.

Examples of the equipment that come under this definition are:
• Patient hoists. (Mobile, ceiling tracking, gantry, bath, standing and bed head.) See Chapter 42, Types of hoist, for more information.
• Slings.
• Stair lifts.

Equipment such as a variable height bed does not come under the regulations as its principal function is as a bed.

A résumé of the regulations is given in Figure 2.1.

In practice, the key issues here are:
• Equipment has to be marked indicating its safe working load.

This means that the handler needs to check the weight of the patient against the safe working load of the hoist and sling. This should be part of the hoist use protocol. It is also important to remember that even if the hoist is able to take the weight of the patient, due to their size and shape it may be necessary to source an alternative hoist and sling.
• Equipment which lifts people to be examined by a competent person at six-monthly intervals.

All hoists should have a sticker on them indicating when they were last serviced and checked and when the next service/check is due. Although it may be the organisation that arranges the servicing schedule, it is the responsibility of the individual handler to check the hoist each time before use.

Provision and Use of Work Equipment Regulations 1998 (PUWER)

The definition of work equipment is 'any machinery appliance, apparatus, tool or installation for the use at work (whether exclusively or not)'.
• A résumé of the regulations is given in Figure 2.2. The instruction 'Ensure work equipment is used for operations for which it is suitable', is the one that is most commonly ignored. An example of this is where a bed sheet is used to move a patient rather than a slide sheet, for example in a lateral transfer (see Chapter 54, 'Transfers from bed to bed/bed to trolley'). Bed sheets are not moving and handling equipment and are not designed for this purpose therefore their use contravenes this regulation.

For clear guidance on the equipment used under LOLER and PUWER please see the HSE website:
www.hse.gov.uk/pubns/hsis4.pdf

Reporting of Injuries, Diseases and Dangerous Occurrences Regulations 2013 (RIDDOR)

A résumé of the regulations is given in Figure 2.3 and full information is available on the HSE website. See link below:
www.hse.gov.uk/riddor/

RIDDOR places responsibilities on employers to report injuries deemed 'reportable' under the act. In relation to back or other musculoskeletal injuries that can happen to patient handlers, Part 4 of the regulation is the one that most commonly applied.

Over-seven-day incapacitation of a worker

Accidents must be reported where they result in an employee or self-employed person being away from work, or unable to perform their normal work duties, for more than seven consecutive days as the result of their injury. This seven-day period does not include the day of the accident, but does include weekends and rest days. The report must be made within 15 days of the accident.

Over-three-day incapacitation

Accidents must be recorded, but not reported where they result in a worker being incapacitated for more than three consecutive days. If you are an employer, who must keep an accident book under the Social Security (Claims and Payments) Regulations 1979, that record will be sufficient.

Human Rights Act 1998

In Figure 2.4, two areas of the Human Rights Act are highlighted.

Article 3: Prohibition of torture

This may not immediately spring to mind as relating to patient handling, but patient handling that is not carried out correctly could be regarded as 'treatment which is inhuman or degrading'. Hoisting a patient with an incorrectly fitting or incorrect type of sling could be termed degrading.

Article 8: Right to respect for home, private and family life

With all aspects of patient handling, the handlers should always be aware of being respectful and maintaining dignity and privacy. The nature of many of the moving and handling tasks means that we may be using equipment to physically move people. It is important to remember the person that is being moved may be anxious or fearful and in an environment that is alien to them.

A short guide on the act is given in:
www.justice.gov.uk/downloads/human-rights/human-rights-making-sense-human-rights.pdf

3 Structure and function of the spine

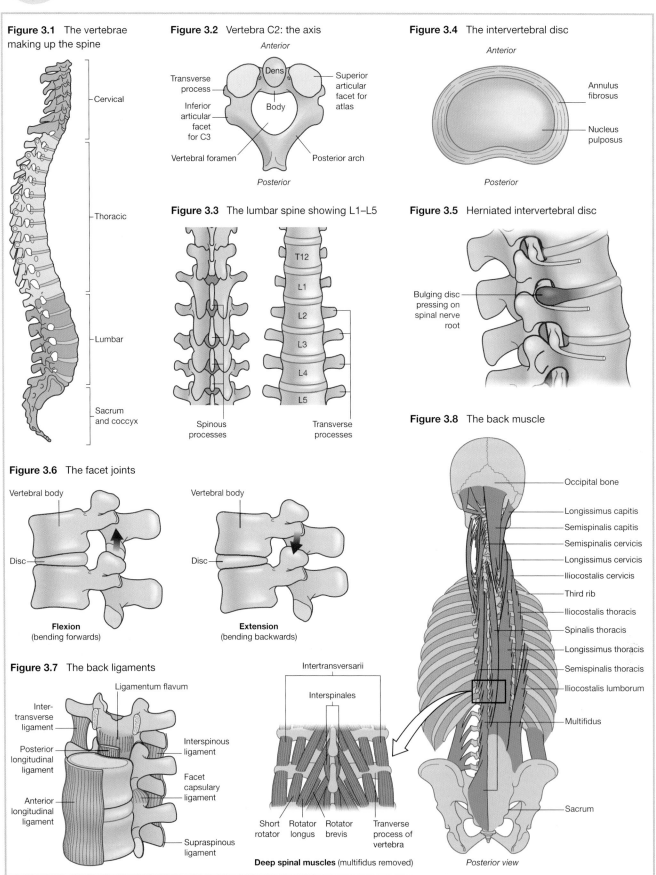

Figure 3.1 The vertebrae making up the spine

- Cervical
- Thoracic
- Lumbar
- Sacrum and coccyx

Figure 3.2 Vertebra C2: the axis

Anterior

Dens
Transverse process
Inferior articular facet for C3
Body
Vertebral foramen
Superior articular facet for atlas
Posterior arch

Posterior

Figure 3.3 The lumbar spine showing L1–L5

T12, L1, L2, L3, L4, L5

Spinous processes

Transverse processes

Figure 3.4 The intervertebral disc

Anterior

Annulus fibrosus
Nucleus pulposus

Posterior

Figure 3.5 Herniated intervertebral disc

Bulging disc pressing on spinal nerve root

Figure 3.6 The facet joints

Vertebral body
Disc

Flexion
(bending forwards)

Vertebral body
Disc

Extension
(bending backwards)

Figure 3.7 The back ligaments

Ligamentum flavum
Inter-transverse ligament
Posterior longitudinal ligament
Anterior longitudinal ligament
Interspinous ligament
Facet capsulary ligament
Supraspinous ligament

Intertransversarii
Interspinales

Short rotator
Rotator longus
Rotator brevis
Tranverse process of vertebra

Deep spinal muscles (multifidus removed)

Figure 3.8 The back muscle

Occipital bone
Longissimus capitis
Semispinalis capitis
Semispinalis cervicis
Longissimus cervicis
Iliocostalis cervicis
Third rib
Iliocostalis thoracis
Spinalis thoracis
Longissimus thoracis
Semispinalis thoracis
Iliocostalis lumborum
Multifidus
Sacrum

Posterior view

Moving and Handling Patients at a Glance. First Edition. Hamish MacGregor. © 2016 John Wiley & Sons, Ltd. Published 2016 by John Wiley & Sons, Ltd.

The spine runs from the base of the skull to the pelvis. It is a double S shape and its main functions are:

- To support the body's weight.
- To protect the spinal cord.

The vertebrae

Thirty-three vertebrae make up the spine and these are divided into four areas (Figure 3.1):

1　The cervical spine (neck) consists of seven vertebrae numbering C1–C7 from top to bottom. Vertebra C1 is also known as the *Atlas* and sits between the skull and the rest of the spine. Vertebra C2, is known as the *Axis*, has a bony projection (odontoid process), the *Dens*, that fits within a hole in the *Atlas* to allow rotation of the neck (Figure 3.2). The remaining cervical vertebrae bend inwards in a C shape and form the cervical lordosis.

2　The thoracic spine consists of 12 vertebrae numbered T1–T12 from top to bottom. The ribs attach to the vertebrae in this section of the spine restricting the range of movement in this area, known as the thoracic kyphosis.

3　The lumbar spine consists of five large vertebrae numbered L1–L5 from top to bottom (Figure 3.3). This area takes the weight of the upper body as well as having a full range of movement. This area, known as the lumbar lordosis.

4　Sacrum and coccyx consist of nine separate segments which are united in the adult so as to form two bones, five entering into the formation of the sacrum, four into that of the coccyx. This is fused and there is no movement. On the whole the sacrum and coccyx are not too problematic as they are fused together. Sometimes if people fall backwards hard they may crack the coccyx.

The intervertebral discs

There are 23 intervertebral discs in the human spine and these are situated between the vertebrae as follows:

- 6 in the cervical spine
- 12 in the thoracic spine
- 5 in the lumbar spine.

　Their function is three-fold:

1　To act as a shock absorber

2　To act as a spacer between the vertebrae

3　To allow movement. Individual disc movement is very limited, however considerable motion is possible when several discs combine forces.

The disc consists of two layers (Figure 3.4): the outer part is the annulus and the inner part the nucleus.

The disc is attached firmly to the vertebra above and below by the ligaments. The disc is oval in shape as it fits on the vertebral body. It is made up of an outer wall (the annulus and an inner nucleus.

The outside wall is made up of 16–20 C-shaped rings of cartilage. They are laid down in opposite directions. This gives the disc good torsional strength.

When you bend forward you place more pressure on the front of the disc. When used correctly it is a good system. Problems occur however when the discs are loaded unevenly. Continued pressure eventually causes the fibres at the back of the disc wall to bulge. This is usually due to the same repeated forces being applied to the same fibres, for example, through repeated bending or through a sudden movement, usually a combination of full forwards and sideways bending. The nucleus works its way through the outside wall and eventually causes the disc to bulge. This is called a slipped disc, prolapsed disc or herniated disc (Figure 3.5). There are no internal nerves in the disc so we are unable to feel this process. However, there are nerves in the very outer layers, so this is when we begin to feel discomfort. Once the bulge presses on surrounding structures that are full of nerves, we feel more severe pain.

The facet joints

The facet joints are like hinges in a dynamic structure which does not lock. They are situated at the back of each vertebra, and they have two key tasks, namely, to allow the spine to bend and twist, and to give the spine stability. When the spine is working well, about 25% of our body weight rests on the facet joints. The facet joints essentially move in three directions forward and backwards (Figure 3.6), sideways and rotation.

Ligaments

The ligaments are tough fibrous connecting tissue that connect the vertebrae (Figure 3.7). Lower back pain is often caused by these ligaments being stretched too far or torn.

Muscles

Back muscles are divided into two specific groups: the extrinsic muscles that are associated with upper extremity and shoulder movement, and the intrinsic muscles that deal with movements of the vertebral column (Figure 3.8).

The extrinsic muscles

Superficial extrinsic muscles connect the upper extremities to the trunk, and they form the V-shaped musculature associated with the middle and upper back. Most of their function is involved with respiration.

The intrinsic muscles

Intrinsic muscles, which stretch all the way from the pelvis to the cranium, help to maintain posture and move the vertebral column. They are divided into three groups: the superficial layer, the intermediate layer, and the deep layer. *Injuries of the intrinsic back muscles often occur while using improper lifting technique. You can protect the back muscles by bending from the hips and knees when you lift objects from the ground.*

Posture and back care

Figure 4.1   Ten top tips for a healthy back

Top 10 tips for a healthy back, including lifting advice, how to sit properly and back-strengthening exercises

1   Exercise your back regularly, walking, swimming (especially backstroke) and using exercise bikes are all excellent ways to strengthen your back muscles.

2   Always bend your knees and hips, not your back.

3   Never twist and bend at the same time.

4   Always lift and carry objects close to your body.

5   Try to carry larger loads in a rucksack, and avoid sling bags.

6   Maintain a good posture. Avoid slouching in your chair, hunching over a desk or walking with your shoulders hunched.

7   Use a chair with a backrest. Sit with your feet flat on the floor or on a footrest. Change how you sit every few minutes.

8   Quit smoking. Smoking reduces the blood supply to the discs between the vertebrae, and this may lead to these discs degenerating.

9   Lose any excess weight.

10   Choose a mattress suited to your height, weight, age and sleeping position.

Reference: http://www.nhs.uk/Livewell/Backpain/Pages/Topbacktips.aspx

Moving and Handling Patients at a Glance. First Edition. Hamish MacGregor. © 2016 John Wiley & Sons, Ltd. Published 2016 by John Wiley & Sons, Ltd.

Posture is the position of your body (including your arms and legs) while you are working. When involved in the moving and handling of patients it is easy to adopt unsafe postures. In many of the following chapters on handling techniques the postures adopted by the handlers show how this can be minimised.

Working with a bent or twisted trunk, raised arms, bent wrists, a bent neck and a turned head increases the risk of back injury and should be avoided, as should twisting, turning and bending movements of the trunk, overreaching, sudden movement and repetitive handling.

Manual handling involves muscular work, of which there are two types:

• Static work: when maintaining a posture (holding the body or part of the body in a fixed position) certain skeletal muscles remain contracted.

• Dynamic work: when moving body parts, active skeletal muscles contract and relax rhythmically.

To use a simple example. If I am carrying a moderately heavy box down a corridor it is my arm muscles that are performing the static work, while my leg muscles carry out dynamic work in walking. It is usually my arm muscles rather than my leg muscles that feel fatigued in this activity.

When working with patients there is a tendency to bend at the waist and lean towards the patient. This is particularly true if the patient is in bed, in a chair or in a wheelchair. This is often referred to as the 'static stoop'. In this posture the joints must be held beyond their comfortable, neutral position and close to the extreme end of their maximum range of movement. If this posture is held for long the handler will become uncomfortable and fatigued. The inter-vertebral discs will be forced into a wedge shape and the disc will bulge out backwards and to the side. See Chapter 3, Structure and function of the spine, for more information.

Achieving a better posture is something that has to be thought about, not just at work but in our day-to-day lives. Try to avoid these postures:

Leaning on one leg, sometimes called 'hanging on one hip'

This position may be adopted when carrying bags over one shoulder and carrying young children on one hip. This can feel comfortable but is often a result of weakness in some muscles and you are placing excessive pressure on one side of your lower back. Over time you can develop muscle imbalances in the pelvis which can lead to low back pain. To improve this posture, stand with your weight distributed evenly between both legs. Exercises to strengthen your buttocks and core muscles will help correct uneven hips.

Sitting with your legs crossed

This puts pressure on your lower back as you are sitting in a slouched position. To correct this:

• Uncross your legs!

• Gently lengthen your neck upwards as you tuck in your chin.

• Pull in your lower stomach muscles to help maintain the natural curve of your lumbar spine.

• Bring your shoulder blades back towards your spine.

Check your seating if you are at a desk. See Chapter 12, Sitting at a desk and workstation set-up, for more information on this. Also see Chapter 13, Postural issues with laptops and tablets.

For more information on improving posture visit the NHS live well website:

www.nhs.uk/Livewell/Backpain/Pages/back-pain-and-common-posture-mistakes.aspx

Be aware of your back

When stretching:

• Stop and think about the movement you are about to make.

• Stretch slowly to reach the object.

• If you cannot reach, do not stretch further.

• Find an alternative way to reach an object such as asking someone for help.

• Use a platform to stand on if the object is high above you or get up and move towards it if it is not within your reach.

When twisting:

• Try to avoid twisting your back at all!

• If you need to reach an object move your feet so that you are facing it.

• Get up to reach an object that is out of your reach.

• NEVER BEND AND TWIST AT THE SAME TIME.

When carrying bags:

• Do not overfill your bag as it can hurt your back by placing a greater load on it.

• Use a rucksack so that the weight is spread over both shoulders.

• Use a smaller bag so that you are not tempted to overfill it.

• Try to find a bag with wheels if you often carry heavy loads.

Finally, try to stay active and healthy:

• See Figure 4.1 for a brief guide.

• Pilates, Yoga and Tai Chi can also help strengthen your back but you must have a *competent* trainer to ensure you are doing this properly.

• If you are in pain seek professional advice as soon as possible.

5 Safe principles of moving and handling

Figure 5.1 Encourage the patient to do as much for themselves as possible

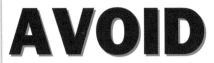

Avoid moving and handling if it at all is practicable to do so.

Figure 5.2 Keeping the spine in line

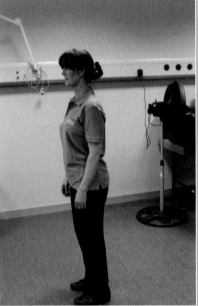

Figure 5.3 Hold loads close to the body

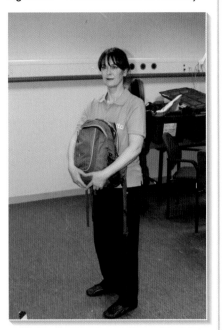

Figure 5.4 Have a stable mobile base with soft flexible knees

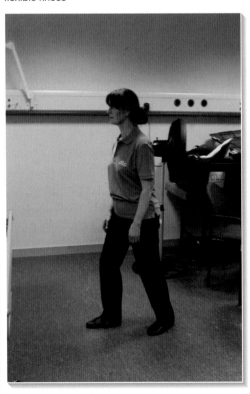

Figure 5.5 Remaining safe principles

- Wear appropriate clothing and footwear.
- Assess the person or object before commencing the handling task.
- Are you competent to carry out this technique?
- If equipment is involved, do you know how to use it?
- Identify a team leader to take charge of the handling task.
- Explain clearly what you are going to do to the patient and obtain their consent.
- Prepare the handling area and ensure it is hazard free.
- Where appropriate apply the brakes on equipment.
- Never twist during a manoeuvre.

Moving and Handling Patients at a Glance. First Edition. Hamish MacGregor. © 2016 John Wiley & Sons, Ltd. Published 2016 by John Wiley & Sons, Ltd.

This section has been divided into two separate parts:

1   Key safe principles of moving and handling.
2   Remaining safe principles of moving and handling.

This in no way suggests a hierarchy of principles but merely a simpler way of tackling the area. The key safe principles in many ways underpin the remaining ones.

Key safe principles

1   **Avoid moving and handling if it is at all practicable to do so.** In relation to patient handling this means encouraging the patient to do as much for themselves as possible (Figure 5.1).

2   **Keeping your spine in line.** This is keeping your spine in its natural curves (see Chapter 2), and keeping your spine in a neutral position. It does not mean that you keep your spine 'poker straight' (Figure 5.2).

3   **Hold the load close.** This is keeping the load, and in some circumstances this may be a patient, as close to your body as possible. As we hold a load away from us it effectively gets heavier. A weight held at arm's length can feel as much as five times as heavy (Figure 5.3).

4   **Having a stable mobile base with soft flexible knees.** Stand with your feet shoulder width apart, one foot slightly in front of the other with soft flexible knees. This allows the handler to transfer their weight back and forth using their quadriceps and gluteal muscles and reduces the pressure on the lower back (Figure 5.4).

Applying the above principles to any handling technique will allow the handler to assess whether the technique is safe or not. If it is unsafe, then it is often possible to see which part of the technique is unsafe and make suitable adjustments.

Remaining safe principles (Figure 5.5)

1   **Wear appropriate clothing and footwear.** The handler must wear loose comfortable clothing so that they are not restricted in any of their movements. The clothing should not be so loose that it causes a hazard by getting caught up in equipment. The same applies to jewellery which can be hazardous and can injure the patient during handling. Footwear should be flat, enclosed, and have a non-slip sole. Footwear such as sandals and flip-flops are never acceptable.

2   **Assess the person or object before commencing a handling task.** Remember that assessment is an ongoing process and needs to be continuously reviewed (see Chapters 7, 8 and 9 for more information).

3   **Are you competent to carry out the technique?** Is your training up to date? Have you had experience in carrying out this technique? Is this a specialist technique that requires additional training and supervision?

4   **If equipment is involved, do you know how to use it?** Have you read the instruction manual? Have you used the equipment recently? If not you may need additional training.

5   **Identify a team leader to take charge of the handling task.** In team handling situations there needs to be a team leader to:
- coordinate the move
- check that all involved are competent to carry out the task
- be the key communicator with the patient, if relevant
- give clear commands
- check that all the handlers are adopting a safe posture.

6   **Explain clearly what you are going to do to the patient and obtain their consent.** The patient needs to be fully cognisant with what is about to happen. Only then will they be able to cooperate fully within their abilities. A patient who does not understand what is happening can be anxious and fearful.

7   **Prepare the handling area and ensure that it is hazard free.** There needs to be enough space to carry out handling tasks; if not, handlers adopt unsafe postures that can lead to cumulative injury. Wet floors can lead to slips and trips. Is there enough lighting to see what you are doing?

8   **Where appropriate apply the brakes on equipment.** Beds, trolleys, commodes and wheelchairs all have brakes that need to be applied appropriately. Remember there are exceptions. Hoist brakes are only used when the hoist is 'parked'. If the brakes are applied when the hoist is in use it may tip over as it cannot move, and therefore find its centre of gravity.

9   **Never twist during a manoeuvre.** This is often difficult to achieve. Remember to move your feet in the direction in which you are moving. This can reduce twisting at the waist by as much as 80%.

6 Controversial techniques

Figure 6.1 The drag lift: the patient is supported underneath the arms

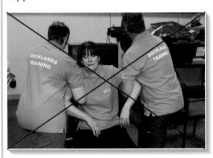

Figure 6.2 The drag lift: with the handlers facing in the opposite direction

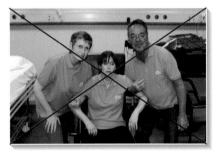

Figure 6.3 The cradle lift

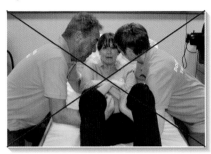

Figure 6.4 The 'bear hug' with the patient's arms around the handler's shoulders

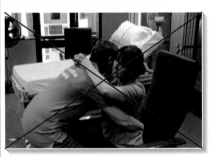

Figure 6.5 Front pivot transfer with the patient's arms around the handler's waist

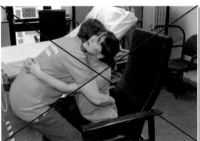
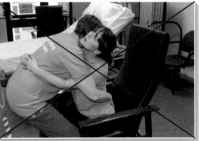

Figure 6.6 Preparing to lift using 'top and tail'

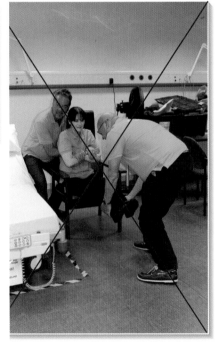

Figure 6.7 Lowering the patient after a 'top and tail' lift

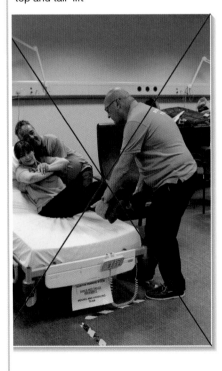

Figure 6.8 Handling equipment should be designed for the purpose

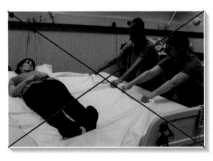

Figure 6.9 A bedsheet should NOT be used as a slide

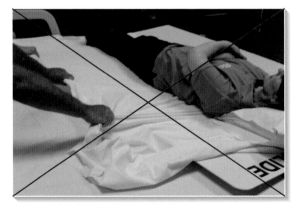

Moving and Handling Patients at a Glance. First Edition. Hamish MacGregor. © 2016 John Wiley & Sons, Ltd. Published 2016 by John Wiley & Sons, Ltd.

ontroversial techniques in the past were known as 'banned techniques' or, incorrectly, 'illegal moves'. These techniques are inherently unsafe for both the patient and the handler and have been ergonomically assessed as being so. Having said this there may be an exceptional circumstance where one of these techniques has to be used, usually in a one-off emergency situation. Should this happen then those involved should complete an incident report under the terms of a 'near miss'. Of course an injury could have actually happened to a handler or the patient and this would constitute the completion of an incident report as an actual injury. It may also lead to the completion of a RIDDOR report. See Chapter 2 for more information on this. If the patient is injured this may be regarded as a safeguarding issue, particularly if it is found to have been unnecessary to move the patient.

After one of these techniques is used there should be a post-analysis of the situation to see if a similar situation arose there could be a safer way of moving the patient.

The harm to the patient is identified below but remember all the techniques present a significant risk to the handler as they cannot apply the safe principles of handling (see Chapter 5).

The techniques

The drag lift (Figures 6.1 and 6.2)

This is where there are two handlers at either side of the patient's bed or chair. The patient is held underneath the arms and dragged up on to the bed or the chair.

Harm to the patient:
- Bruising on the arm.
- Sublaxation of the shoulder joint.
- Brachial plexus damage.
- Fracture of the humerus.
- Pain.
- Tissue viability problems especially to the heels, sacrum and shoulder blades.
- The patient is immobilised and apart from possibly digging their heels into the bed cannot assist in the technique.

Orthodox or cradle lift (Figure 6.3)

This is where there are two handlers at either side of the patient's bed or chair. The patient is held behind their back and under their thighs, and is lifted up on to the bed or chair.

Harm to the patient:
- Pain.
- Tissue viability problems especially to the heels, sacrum and shoulder blades.
- Bruising where the handler is holding the patient.
- As both handlers are picking the patient up like a child, there are dignity issues for the patient.
- The patient is immobilised and cannot participate in the manoeuvre.

Bear hug (Figure 6.4)

This is where the handler stands in front of the chair and allows the patient to put their arms around the handler's neck. The handler then stands the patient.

Harm to the patient:
- The patient cannot participate in the manoeuvre as the handler is standing in front of them and therefore blocking natural body movement, i.e. the patient cannot get their nose over their toes.
- The patient may fall as both they and the handler are unsteady.
- As the patient's arms are around the handler's neck they are unable to push up from the chair with their arms, leading to unsteadiness.

Front pivot transfer (Figure 6.5)

This is similar to the bear hug, but the patient's arms are around the handler's waist. This technique, once the patient is out of the chair, results in the patient being pivoted around onto another chair, bed or commode.

Harm to the patient:
- The patient cannot participate in the manoeuvre as the handler is standing in front of them and therefore blocking natural body movement, i.e. the patient cannot get their nose over their toes.
- The patient may fall as both they and the handler are unsteady.
- The patient cannot move their feet and are therefore more likely to fall.
- The handler may fall on top of the patient and injure them.

Top and tail (Figures 6.6 and 6.7)

The patient is in a chair and is to be transferred to a bed. One handler is at the top of the patient with their arms under the patient's arm pits, and their hands are crossed over the patient's chest. The second handler is at the patient's feet/legs. The two handlers then lift (and throw) the patient from the chair to the bed.

Harm to the patient:
- Bruising on the arm and legs and hips.
- Sublaxation of the shoulder joint.
- Brachial plexus damage.
- Fracture of the humerus.
- Fracture to ribs.
- Pain.
- Fear.
- Loss of dignity for the patient, as the handler at the patient's head ends up in the bed with the patient.

Using equipment not designed for the purpose (Figures 6.8 and 6.9)

The usual example of this is using a bed sheet to move a patient on a PAT slide.

Harm to the patient:
- Tissue viability problems as there is increased friction when using a sheet instead of a slide sheet.
- The sheet may tear causing the patient to be injured.

Using 1, 2, 3 as a command

The main injury here is to the handler as they do not know whether to move on 3 or the imaginary 4. But as the patient can be unclear when to move, they can be injured too. It is often better to use 'Ready, Steady…' than an action word such as 'Stand'.

Risk assessment: moving and handling

Figure 7.1 The six component parts in a moving and handling risk assessment: 1. The task. 2. The individual capability. 3. The (a) load or (b) person. 4. The environment. 5. The equipment that is being used. 6. Other influencing factors.

1. Task

Factors that may need to be considered:

- Can you apply the key safe principles of handling (see Chapter 5)?
- Be aware of static postures (see Chapter 4).
- Can you avoid twisting?
- Do you need to carry over a long distance?
- Are there unpredictable movements of loads?
- Does this involve repetitive handling?
- Are there sufficient breaks factored into the task?

2. Individual capability

Factors that may need to be considered:

Does the job:

- Require a certain level of fitness?
- Present a risk to those who have pre-existing health problems?
- Constitute a hazard to those who are pregnant?
- Require specialised training?
- Require a certain level of knowledge, skills and competency?
- Become more risky at certain times of the day?

3. (a) Load

Factors that may need to be considered:

Are the loads:

- Heavy?
- Bulky?
- Difficult to grasp?
- Unstable or have an uneven weight distribution?
- Potentially harmful, for example hot?

(b) Person

Factors that may need to be considered:

In relation to handling people, many of the previous *load* factors can be applied to *people*.

In addition we need to consider:

- Medical conditions that will affect handling.
- Level of understanding?
- Level of cooperation?
- Conscious level.
- Pain.
- Attachments: intravenous lines, catheters, drains, etc.

4. Environment

Factors that may need to be considered:

- Is there enough space?
- Type of flooring?
- Are there stairs to be negotiated?
- Is there a good ergonomic layout?
- Are there obstacles in the way?
- Is the temperature conducive to the work being carried out?
- Is there sufficient lighting?

5. The equipment that is being used

Factors that may need to be considered:

- Is it appropriate for the task?
- Has the safe working load been identified?
- Is it in good working order and free from damage?
- Has it been serviced/checked in accordance with legal requirements, for example LOLER? (see Chapter 2)
- Do the staff require any special training to operate the equipment?

6. Other influencing factors

- Levels of stress or other psychosocial factors.
- Poor staffing levels or staffing levels supplemented by high numbers of agency staff.
- Pressures of work or at home.
- Organisational policies.

Moving and Handling Patients at a Glance. First Edition. Hamish MacGregor. © 2016 John Wiley & Sons, Ltd. Published 2016 by John Wiley & Sons, Ltd.

There are six component parts in a moving and handling risk assessment:

- The task
- The individual capability
- The load or person
- The environment
- The equipment that is being used
- Other influencing factors.

All of the above are described in Figure 7.1. Please read through the section opposite first. There are some expanded sections below that look at some risk-reducing measures that can be adopted. These are purely illustrative and are not meant to be a comprehensive list.

Task

The application of the safe principles of moving and handling is fundamental to any moving and handling task (see Chapter 5). If you are unable to keep your spine in line, the load close and adopt a mobile stable base with soft flexible knees, then the task is inherently unsafe. Thought needs to be given to areas such as:

- Task redesign
- Introduction of equipment
- Increase in staffing level
- Re-training staff.

The hazards of adopting poor postures, particularly the static stoop, can contribute significantly to cumulative injury (see Chapter 4).

When you find yourself moving objects over long distances, use trolleys so that you are pushing rather than lifting. If this is not possible, are there points at which you can put down your load so that you can have a rest before continuing?

In relation to unpredictable loads, this can apply to both inanimate objects and people.

Moving a water bottle onto a cooler is difficult in many ways, but especially as it is lifted the water moves around and the centre of gravity changes all the time. Risk-reducing measures include using smaller bottles, having the water bottles stored at shelf height next to the cooler, using two people and ultimately having a plumbed in system that negates the need to move the bottles at all.

People when they are being moved should be comprehensively assessed so that the unpredictability factor is reduced. Someone who is small but confused and unable to understand instructions can pose a higher risk to staff than a very large patient who is able to cooperate fully with staff.

Individual capability

All individuals who handle loads and/or people are different, therefore the handlers are a key element of the risk assessment process.

We all have different levels of fitness and stamina that affect our ability to perform throughout the day.

Due to the cumulative effects on those who carry out handling tasks, we need to be aware that some of our colleagues may have pre-existing back problems. This may require seeking help from Occupational Health and adjustments made to their work, either on a temporary or permanent basis.

Staff may have varying levels of skills and competence when carrying out moving and handling tasks. Factors that need to be addressed are:

Training that they have received. When was it? What was the content? Was it relevant to their current role? Did they have an opportunity to practise any techniques taught? Was there an opportunity to ask questions? Did the training address the learning styles of the learner? Was the learners' competency assessed? Did the learners receive constructive feedback?

All of the above factors may help in addressing any further training input that may be needed.

Certain times of the day may make injury to staff more likely. At the end of a busy working week this may increase. Many nursing staff work long days which may contribute to fatigue, which can in turn lead to an increase in musculo-skeletal injury.

Load or person

The Manual Handling Operation Regulations (1992) give us guidelines for when an inanimate load needs to be risk assessed based on weight and its position in relation to the body. See Chapter 10, Lifting a load, for more details.

People are complex; therefore remember there are no safe working loads.

When looking at factors such as the weight, size or shape of a person we can reduce risk by:

- Having appropriate equipment at hand
- Specialised training
- Increase in staffing.

Many of the complicating factors with people handling are not to do with the size/shape of the person, but relate to communication issues. Therefore we need to use:

- Translation services if required
- Well-developed skills in communicating with people who may have cognitive problems, dysphasia or hearing problems.

Many patients' medical conditions will require the handler to have a suitable knowledge of that condition and how it can affect the patient's mobility.

Examples of this would be:

- Parkinson's disease
- Stroke
- Multiple sclerosis
- Patients with painful conditions.

Environment

In assessing the environment it is important to identify the hazards and consider if they affect people's posture or present a slip, trip or fall hazard. Then it may be necessary to:

- Move equipment to another place.
- Create better storage areas.
- Increase the lighting.
- Increase the number of warning signs.
- Monitor temperature levels.

Equipment that is being used

Consider:

- An equipment audit to take stock of what is in place, its condition, age and suitability.
- Planned replacement programme for older equipment.
- Are servicing contracts suitable and sufficient?
- Competency levels of staff using the equipment.

Other influencing factors

In looking at the factors mentioned in Figure 7.1 try to think broadly about any other factors that may be relevant in the risk reduction process.

8 Risk assessment: general

Figure 8.1 Risk assessment matrix

Likelihood of recurrence	Consequence of incident				
	Insignificant (1)	Minor (2)	Moderate (3)	Major (4)	Catastrophic (5)
Almost certain (5)	5	10	15	20	25
Likely (4)	4	8	12	16	20
Possible (3)	3	6	9	12	15
Unlikely (2)	2	4	6	8	10
Rare (1)	1	2	3	4	5

Notes:

Almost certain (5), will probably occur frequently

Likely (4), will probably occur, but not as a persistent issue

Possible (3), may occur

Unlikely (2), not expected to occur

Rare (1), would only occur in exceptional circumstances

Figure 8.2 Consequence: outcome of the incident in terms of harm

Descriptor	Risk consequence score			
	Injury/harm	Service delivery	Financial	Reputation/publicity
Catastrophic (5)	Unanticipated death/large number injured or affected (e.g. breast screening errors).	Breakdown/closure of a critical service	£5M	• Long-term/repeated adverse national publicity that undermines patient and/or referrer confidence • Chair/CEO and/or executive team removal
Major (4)	Major permanent loss of function (for a patient unrelated to natural course of illness/underlying condition/pregnancy/childbirth).	Intermittent failures in a critical service	£1M – £5M	• Widespread and sustained adverse publicity • Increased level of political/public scrutiny
Moderate (3)	Semi-permanent harm (1 month–1 year). >1 month's absence from work for staff.	Sustained period of disruption to services	£100k – £1M	Widespread or high profile adverse publicity
Minor (2)	Short-term injury (<1 month). 3 days to 1 month's absence for staff.	Short disruption to services that affects patient care	£10k – £100k	Adverse publicity
Insignificant (1)	Minor harm. Injury resulting in < 7 days' absence from work for staff.	Service disruption that does not affect patient care	<£10k	None

Moving and Handling Patients at a Glance. First Edition. Hamish MacGregor. © 2016 John Wiley & Sons, Ltd. Published 2016 by John Wiley & Sons, Ltd.

The need to carry out moving and handling risk assessments is outlined in the Manual Handling Operations Regulations (1992) as amended in 2002 (see Chapter 1 for more details). The regulations state that we should assess any hazardous manual handling operations that cannot be avoided. The purpose of this is to reduce the risk of injury to the lowest level reasonably practicable.

Definition of risk

A risk assessment is a careful examination of what could cause harm to people, so that you can weigh up whether you have taken enough precautions or should do more to prevent harm.

It is important to understand the terms hazard and risk.

- A hazard is anything that may cause harm;
- A risk is the chance or likelihood that harm will occur.

The Health and Safety executive (HSE) talks of *five steps to risk assessment.*

Step 1: Identify the hazards

- How can people be harmed?
- Look around your workplace and identify the hazards.
- Ask others who work in the area to assist. They may notice things that you do not.
- Checking manufacturer's instructions of equipment can help you in identifying the hazards.
- Look at the number of incidents and near misses.

Step 2: Decide who might be harmed and how

- For each hazard you need to identify who might be harmed, not only individuals but also groups of people.
- Groups of people could be staff, patients, visitors, contactors, etc.
- Be aware that some staff are more at risk than others, for example staff who have pre-existing injures or who are pregnant.

Step 3: Evaluate the risks and decide on precautions

- Having spotted the hazards then you have to plan what you are going to do about them. The law states that you need to do everything 'reasonably practicable' to protect people from harm.
- Look carefully at what is happening at present. Are there some existing controls in place?

- Compare what is happening with identified good practice elsewhere.
- Can the hazards be removed completely? If not, how are you going to reduce them?
- When evaluating the risk it is useful to look at the consequence of the event happening, then look at the likelihood of it happening. You can plot this on a matrix that will give you a risk rating. An example is given in Figure 8.1.

Step 4: Record your findings and implement them

- Document the results of your findings. Your documentation must have an action plan.
- Keep the results simple. It is important to prioritise and tackle the most harmful risks first. This is where the use of the matrix in Figure 8.2 can be useful.
- It is often useful to list your findings on a scale beginning with the simple easily achievable ones with little or no budgetary implications through to the more complex ones with bigger budgetary implications.
- If there are things that are more complex escalate them through the management of the organisation to ensure they are examined at the correct level.
- You may have to put in temporary solutions where the ideal risk-reducing measure is not immediately achievable.

Step 5: Review your risk assessment and update if necessary

- Few workplaces stay the same. Sooner or later, you will bring in new equipment and procedures that could lead to new hazards. It makes sense, therefore, to review what you are doing on an ongoing basis. Every year or so formally review where you are, to make sure you are still improving, or at least not sliding back.
- Look at your risk assessment again. Have there been any changes?
- Are there improvements you still need to make?
- Have the staff spotted a problem?
- Have you learnt anything from accidents or near misses?
- Make sure your risk assessment stays up to date. Set a review date when you complete the assessment. If there is a change in the intervening time then you need to go back and check it and make any amendments as are necessary.

Remember the risk assessment process is a dynamic one which needs to flexible enough to meet the ever changing needs of the workplace.

Individual patient handling assessment

Figure 9.1 Individual patient handling assessment form

Please complete or affix label
Surname: *Mrs Patient*

Forename: *Josephine*

Date of Birth: *12th October 1945*

Ward:_____ *One* _____

Sheet No:_____

INDIVIDUAL PATIENT HANDLING ASSESSMENT

Is patient totally independent? ■/No*
If Yes: assessment need go no further Assessor's signature_____ Print Name_____
          Designation _____ Date_____ Review date_____ Reason for review_____
If No: Continue the assessment   * **delete as necessary**

Weight (kg): *58.1kg*	Height (cm): *1.71*	Risk of falls: High/■*

Any problems with comprehension, behaviour, cooperation? E.g., hearing, speech, language barriers, unpredictable, depressed, behavioural problems, poor motivation
She is unable to talk, but opens eyes and nods for 'yes' and shakes her head for 'no'. She has movement in her right hand and can use the bed controls.

Handling constraints? E.g., conscious/unconscious, disability, weakness, pain, skin lesions, spasticity, attachment to equipment, joint replacement, balance, ability to weight bear, mobility
Dependent. Flexor spasm in her lower limbs. Catheter

Other problems:
She has lived in supported accommodation for 3 years
Refer to Moving and Handling Advisor? Yes/■ ■*

SAFE SYSTEM OF WORK

Handling task	Independent ✓	Supervised ✓	Hoist ✓	Assistance no of carers	Explain how to do procedure and equipment required, e.g., transfer board, patslide, slide sheets, electric profiling bed, bath aids, shower chair
Turning/ Rolling In bed		✓		2	*To reposition for pressure relief. Two flat slide sheets inserted from head of bed, roll on side using slide sheets with a minimum of two staff*
Lying to sitting		✓		1	*Electric profiling bed*
Up/down the bed		✓		2	*Two flat slide sheets, insert from head of bed. Remove bedhead and pull from head of bed*
Sitting to standing					*Not applicable*
Bed to chair or commode chair to bed or commode			✓	2	*Arjo Maximove hoist, disposable medium high back sling, insert as per training on one roll. Pillows to support her in recliner chair*
Walking					*Not applicable*
Toileting In or out of bed (specify which toilet)			✓	2	*Hoist to commode.*
Bath or shower (specify which room)			✓	2	*Large bathroom. Hoist from bed to bathroom. Adjust height of bath as protocol. Or wash in bed.*
Bed to trolley transfers		✓		3	*Patslide, three flat slide sheets. Four extension handles. Procedure as per protocol.*

Assessor's Signature__ *AM Busy* _____ Print Name__ *AM BUSY* _____

Designation__ *SN* _____ Time__ *10.30 a.m.* _____ Date *7th February 2015* _____

Proposed date of review: *14th Feb 15* _____ Reason for review_ *Change in medical condition* _____

Why record the assessment?

The law requires us to complete assessments in order to reduce the risk of injury to the lowest level reasonably practicable.

The assessment should reduce this risk of injury for the patients and all handlers.

The completion of such an assessment should raise awareness of any handling constraints the patient may have.

If there is an accident or a near miss related to the patient's handling needs, then an assessment can show that you acted according to your best judgement at the time.

Note: Please refer to Chapter 7 on risk assessment if you have not already done so.

Do not attempt an assessment on a patient if you do not have the knowledge and skills to do so. Seek help and advice.

An example of an Individual Patient Handling Assessment is on the page opposite (Table 9.1). Here is some guidance on its completion.

The top two boxes of the assessment form, need to be completed fully prior to the assessment to ensure this applies to the correct patient.

Is the patient totally independent? Yes/No.

If yes, the assessment should go no further. This must be completed, signed and dated even if the patient has no handling needs at that time. This proves that an assessment has been carried out. Remember a patient may come into hospital independent, but this may change postoperatively.

If no then the assessment needs to be completed.

Recording the assessment

• Clear statements of the patient's abilities should be used and all handling constraints listed.
• Reassess if significant effort is required to achieve a transfer.
• Refer to existing protocols from generic assessments to save writing out details, if they apply to this patient.

• Select techniques that encourage patient independence, or use appropriate handling equipment. Do not use controversial techniques (see Chapter 6).
• Instructions should be clear and with relevant information to allow the manoeuvre to be carried out safely.
• Seek advice if a safe solution cannot be identified.
• Interim control measures must be identified if relevant equipment is not immediately available, for example appropriate hoist.
• If, when about to carry out a transfer there are new problems, or changes in the patient's abilities which differ from the assessment, **STOP,** reassess or refer to patient's nurse/physiotherapist/occupational therapist/family, etc.
• Evaluate the task routinely after it has been completed. If necessary update the form.

Selecting a technique

Having considered existing written procedures and their relevance to this patient's specific abilities and needs, the assessor must decide on one of a number of ways to carry out the task:
• Let the patient move themselves
• Use a mechanical device
• Use a sliding system
• Do not do the task.

Decisions regarding these choices should be made following adequate moving and handling training. If you are unsure of how to work safely, advice should be sought from your manager or the moving and handling advisor.

Evaluation after handling the patient

Once the task has been completed, it should be immediately evaluated. This only needs to be an informal process, but it should be gone through conscientiously to ensure that handling remains safe.

Evaluation

Table 9.1 Individual Patient Handling Assessment

Consider:	Then:	Action:
Has the patient's condition improved?	Is there sufficient improvement to allow the patient to contribute more to the task?	If yes: the task should be reassessed
Has the patient's condition deteriorated?	Is the patient still able to contribute the required effort?	If no: the task should be reassessed
What was the patient's reaction to the technique?	Did the patient resist the move? Did he feel uncomfortable or disorientated in any way?	If problems were experienced the task needs to be reassessed
Did all those involved in the task carry out their roles correctly?		If no: either the person needs retraining or the task should be reassessed
Did the equipment work correctly?		Report equipment failures immediately and withdraw it from use
Did the equipment perform as expected?		If no: the task should be reassessed or staff must be retrained in its use

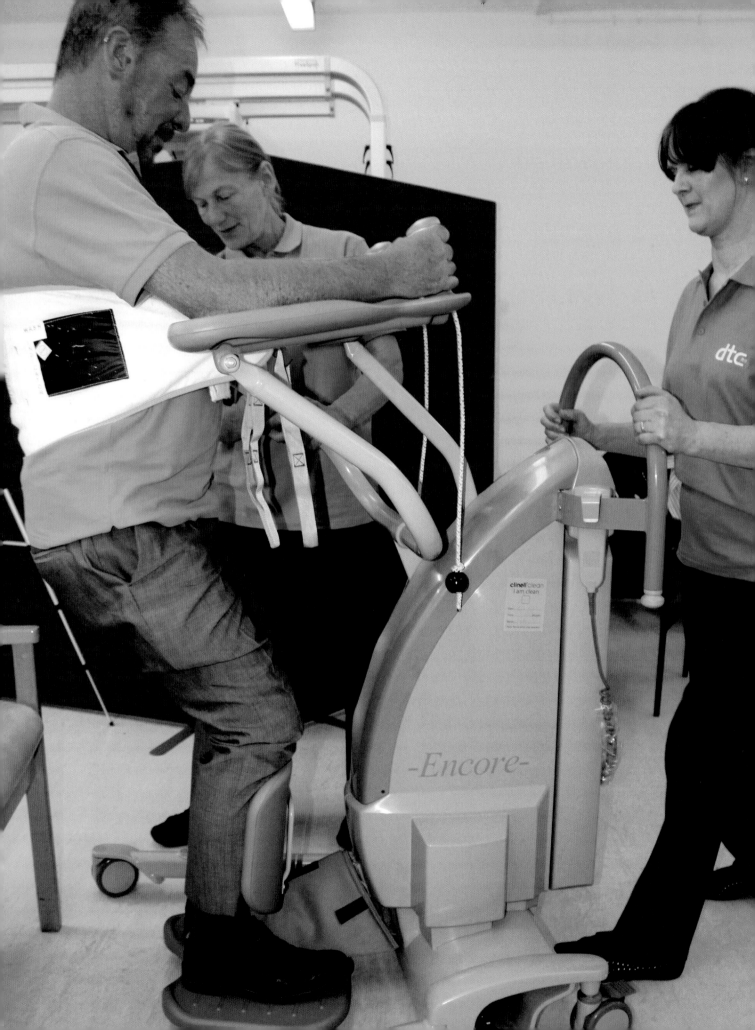

Practice

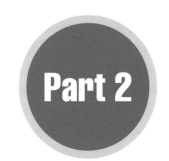
Part 2

Chapters

10 Lifting a load

Figure 10.1 The maximum weight that can be safely lifted by male and female handlers before a risk assessment should be carried out.

Source: Published by the Health and Safety Executive and licensed under the Open Government Licence.

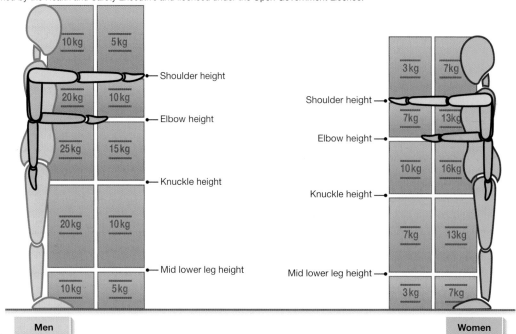

Men:
- Shoulder height: 10 kg / 5 kg
- Elbow height: 20 kg / 10 kg
- Knuckle height: 25 kg / 15 kg
- Mid lower leg height: 20 kg / 10 kg
- (floor): 10 kg / 5 kg

Women:
- Shoulder height: 3 kg / 7 kg
- Elbow height: 7 kg / 13 kg
- Knuckle height: 10 kg / 16 kg
- Mid lower leg height: 7 kg / 13 kg
- (floor): 3 kg / 7 kg

Figure 10.2 Move the box close before attempting to lift it

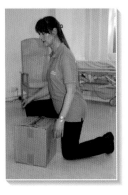

Figure 10.3 Get a good hold on the box and slide it up the thigh

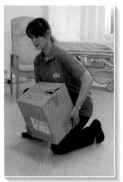

Figure 10.4 Move the box onto the thigh of the opposite leg

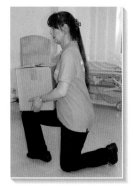

Figure 10.5 Move the box to waist height, keeping it close to the body

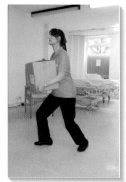

Figure 10.6 Move to face the place where the box will be deposited

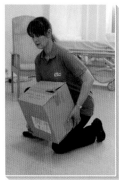

Figure 10.7 Lower the box by bending at the hips and knees

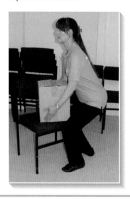

Figure 10.8 Slide the box safely onto the surface

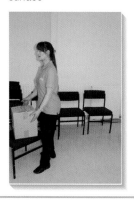

Moving and Handling Patients at a Glance. First Edition. Hamish MacGregor. © 2016 John Wiley & Sons, Ltd. Published 2016 by John Wiley & Sons, Ltd.

Purpose

To move a load safely whilst maintaining a good posture

Before the manoeuvre

1   Is there a written risk assessment in place covering this manoeuvre?
2   Assess the environment and ensure there are no obstacles.
3   Assess the load by checking the weight, shape, size and contents of the box. In assessing the contents of the box look at areas such as:
   • Distribution of weight.
   • Are the contents likely to shift?
   • Are they potentially harmful?
   • Are the contents likely to spill?
4   Are you fit to carry out the manoeuvre?
5   Do you need assistance?
6   Do you require equipment to carry out the task?
7   Check the position of the box in relation to the height that it is stored in relation to your body. The Manual Handling Operations Regulations (1992) as amended in 2002 give guidelines for lifting and lowering. These guidelines give the maximum weight that can be lifted in ideal conditions by a man or woman before a suitable and sufficient risk assessment is carried out. This is dependent on the position of the load (high or low) and the distance from the body (Figure 10.1). If we take the example of the handler here in Figure 10.2, the maximum load she can move from the floor, as the box is close to her, is 7 kg. This guidance is only applied to inanimate objects and *does not apply to people*. See Chapter 7, Risk assessment, for more information.

During the manoeuvre

1   Bend down to the box with one knee on the floor and keep your spine in line. Move the box close to you by getting one corner to point towards you (Figure 10.2).
2   Get a good hand hold on the box and slide the box up the thigh of the leg that is kneeling on the floor (Figure 10.3).
3   Move the box onto the thigh of the opposite leg. You may find it necessary to have a rest here before continuing with the manoeuvre (Figure 10.4).
4   Moving the box to waist height, stand up keeping the box close you at all times (Figure 10.5).
5   Turn to face where the box is to be placed (in this case, a chair, which has been correctly positioned prior to movement). Move your feet in the direction in which you are going. Avoid twisting from the waist (Figure 10.6).
6   Bending at the hips and knees, lower the box to the chair. Always keep the box close to your body. Keep your head up (Figure 10.7).
7   Do not be tempted to hold the box away from you as it is lowered onto the chair. If necessary slide the box away from you once it is on the chair (Figure 10.8).

Other factors to consider

1   If the surface of the box has sharp edges, or is hot or dirty, then consider using protective clothing such as gloves and aprons.
2   Very large and bulky objects may not be heavy, but can be difficult to move as you may not be able to see over them, so this may prelude your carrying out the technique.

11 Pushing a bed

Figure 11.1   The brake in the 'On' position

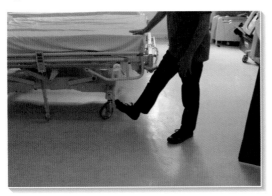

Figure 11.2   The brake in the 'Steer' position

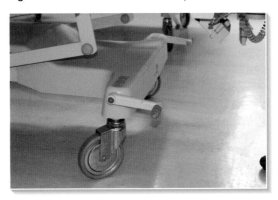

Figure 11.3   The brake in the 'Free wheel' position

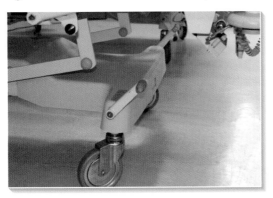

Figure 11.4   Bed raised to a good height for the handler

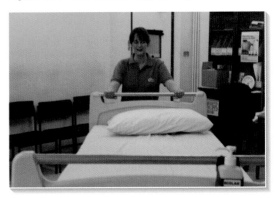

Figure 11.5   Adopt a step stance position before pushing the bed

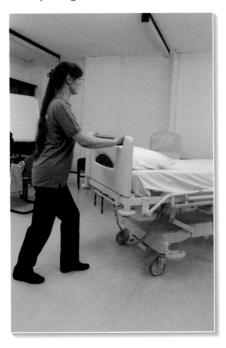

Figure 11.6   Using hips and thighs move the bed slowly

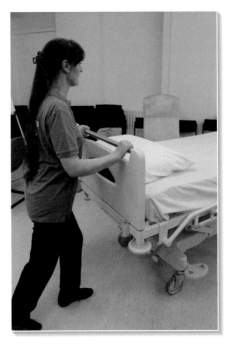

Moving and Handling Patients at a Glance. First Edition. Hamish MacGregor. © 2016 John Wiley & Sons, Ltd. Published 2016 by John Wiley & Sons, Ltd.

Purpose

To move a bed safely from one destination to another. The principles of this manoeuvre can be applied to most situations where it is necessary to push an object.

Before the move

1   Be cognisant with local policies and procedure that will dictate how many people should move a bed and in what circumstances.

2   Check that there is a clear path for you to move the bed, free from any obstacles.

3   Ensure that you are fit enough to move the bed; you may need to enlist help.

4   Know how the brake/steer controls of the bed work.
  • Brake (Figure 11.1).
  • Steer (Figure 11.2). This allows the bed to be pushed in a straight line as two wheels are locked in a forwards position.
  • Freewheel (Figure 11.3). All four wheels move freely. This is good for small manoeuvres into bed spaces, etc. This means it is difficult to control the direction of the bed and if you are on your own moving the bed, twisting of the lower back and potential injury may occur. A second handler should assist here at all times.

5   If the bed head and foot are not on the bed, they should be attached as this will give the handler a good handhold to manoeuvre the bed.

6   If this is an electric bed, unplug it before you move the bed and ensure that the plug and flex are secure so as not to trail on the floor during the move.

During the manoeuvre

1   Move to the head of the bed.

2   With the bed raised to a height that allows the handler to adopt a good posture, place your hands on the bed-head (Figure 11.4).

3   Adopting a step stance position with your spine in line, get ready to push the bed (Figure 11.5).

4   Pushing from the hips and thighs start to move the bed slowly. This needs to be a slow controlled move with no jerky movements (Figure 11.6).

Other factors to consider

1   If a patient is in the bed then you need to be fully cognisant with local policies and protocols about number of staff and their roles in pushing the patient and caring for the patient.

2   If the patient is in the bed then side rails or transport sides will need to be raised. Ensure that you do not take hold of the side rails to steer the bed, as they are not designed for the purpose.

3   If a patient is in the bed and they are on a low air loss mattress, then ensure that it is in transport mode before moving the bed so that the mattress does not deflate during the journey.

4   If the bed is a specialist bed, for example, a bariatric bed, then it will need more people to move the bed due to its increased size and weight.

5   When pushing beds through doors, if they are not slow closing or have magnetic door holders, you will need another person to hold the doors open.

12 Good workstation set-up

Figure 12.1 Good sitting posture for computer

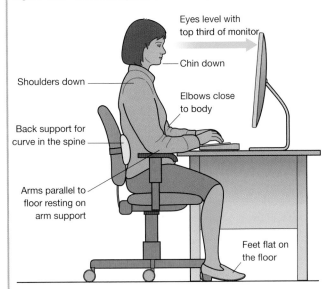

- Eyes level with top third of monitor
- Chin down
- Shoulders down
- Elbows close to body
- Back support for curve in the spine
- Arms parallel to floor resting on arm support
- Feet flat on the floor

Figure 12.2 Use of a lumbar support

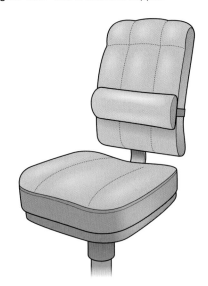

Figure 12.3 Using a variable height desk

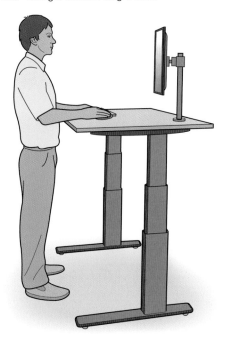

Figure 12.4 Keep things within easy reach

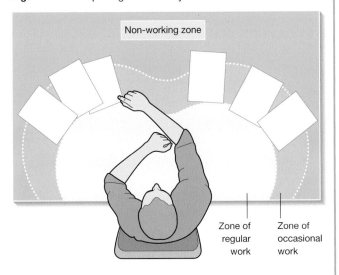

- Non-working zone
- Zone of regular work
- Zone of occasional work

Figure 12.6 Example of a vertical mouse

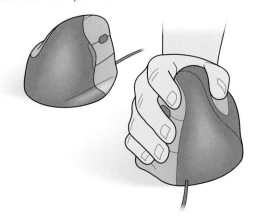

Figure 12.5 Use a mouse mat with a wrist support

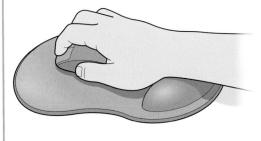

Moving and Handling Patients at a Glance. First Edition. Hamish MacGregor. © 2016 John Wiley & Sons, Ltd. Published 2016 by John Wiley & Sons, Ltd.

Sitting at a computer for long periods of time can cause neck, shoulder and back problems. To minimise this there are a number of things that need to be addressed.

Workstation set-up

Your chair

The more that you can adjust the chair the better chance you will have to achieve a good ergonomic posture.

Basically you are hoping to keep your upper and lower limbs at approximately 90 degrees (Figure 12.1). It is often useful to have the seat tilted forward; this means that your hips are higher than your knees and you are taking some weight through your legs. If you have a pre-existing back problem you must check with a health professional (for example, a physiotherapist) if this is suitable for you.

Your feet need to be flat on the floor. If this is not possible you need a footrest.

Adjust the depth of the seat to allow for a space of about four fingers width between the edge of the seat and the back of your knees.

The back rest needs to be adjusted to give support of your lumbar curve. If your chair has an inflatable lumbar support, this is ideal. If you have a large lumbar curve, it may be necessary to use a lumbar support (Figure 12.2).

If the chair has a free float mechanism that allows you to move in the chair, then do not lock it. This will allow you to move in the chair and this is an important part of reducing back injury.

If there are arm rests on the chair, they need to be adjusted so that the elbows are supported with your shoulders relaxed. The arm rests should not prevent you from getting closer to your desk.

Your desk

A desk that is too low can cause you to adopt a C-shaped spine. A desk that is too high can cause pressure on your shoulders and lead to neck pain.

The ideal desk height allows you (once you have set up your chair correctly) to have your elbows parallel with your keyboard and your forearms parallel to the floor (Figure 12.1).

A sit to stand desk (Figure 12.3) can allow you to alternate between sitting and standing and reduce the risk of continuous static postures; this promotes good back health.

Your work top

Set up your desk surface so that you can reach the things that you use most without stretching. This is the keyboard, but also your mouse and possibly a phone (Figure 12.4).

The monitor should be about an arm's length away, with your eyes facing the top third of the screen. If there is a problem seeing the screen, professional advice needs to be sought. Some people have glasses that are specifically to be used with their computer.

Your mouse should have a mouse mat with a wrist support (Figure 12.5). This will allow the wrist to be kept in a neutral position. If you are experiencing wrist, hand or shoulder problems, seek help before it becomes a problem. The use of an alternative type of mouse such as a vertical mouse (Figure 12.6) or roller-ball mouse may help alleviate the problem. Learn keyboard shortcuts, which will reduce the need for you to use your mouse. Try to learn to use your mouse with both hands, thus reducing strain on your dominant side.

General problems

Laptops

See Chapter 13 for more information.

Hot desking

Remember to take a few minutes to adjust your workstation to your needs before you start work.

Sitting at the workstation for too long a time

Take frequent breaks. Ideally you should not sit at a computer for more than 20 minutes. If you get into the habit of getting up and stretching on a regular basis this will help your back.

Useful resources

There are a number of leaflets that can help address the issues mentioned above, and there are some resources produced by Backcare, the charity for back and neck pain:

Setting up your workstation

www.backcare.org.uk/wp-content/uploads/2015/02/Setting-up-your-Workstation-Factsheet.pdf

Exercises for office workers

www.backcare.org.uk/wp-content/uploads/2015/01/703-Eurocrat-220910.pdf

Choosing a chair

www.backcare.org.uk/wp-content/uploads/2015/01/107-Eurocrat-210910.pdf

Office furniture

www.backcare.org.uk/wp-content/uploads/2015/01/102-Eurocrat-210910.pdf

The legal position

The Health and Safety (Display Screen Equipment) Regulation 1992 applies to employers whose workers regularly use DSE as a significant part of their normal work (daily, for continuous periods of an hour or more). Although this is not likely to apply to the readers of this book, it does give some useful guidance and covers areas such as assessing workstations, putting controls in place, providing information and training and having reviews of assessments as changes take place. See Working with Display Screen Equipment (DSE).

A brief guide: www.hse.gov.uk/pubns/indg36.pdf

13 Postural issues with laptops and tablets

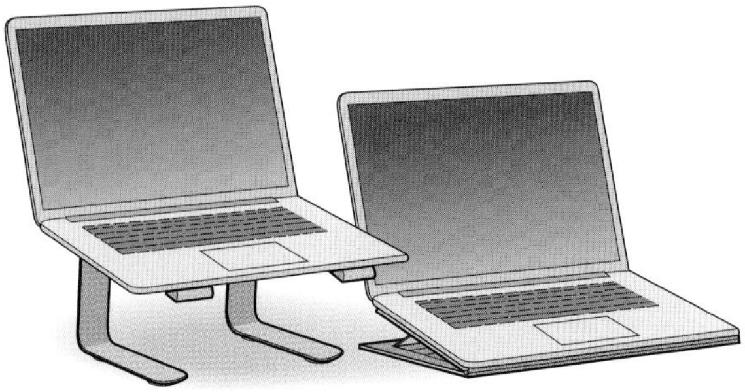

Figure 13.1 Examples of laptop stands

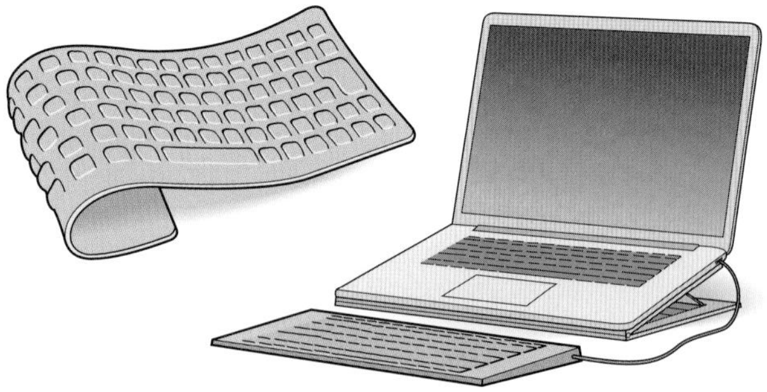

Figure 13.2 Examples of keyboards

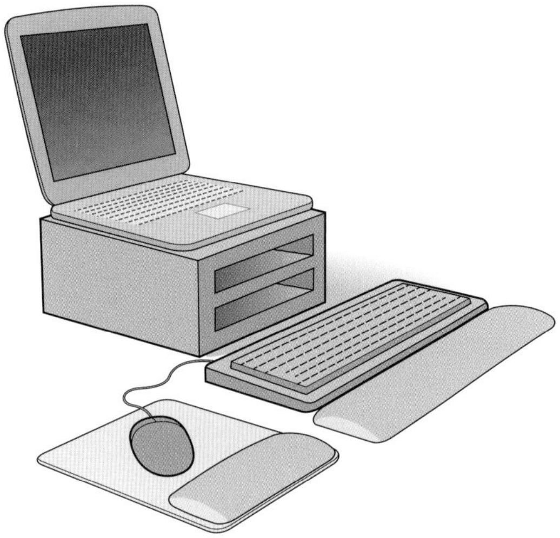

Figure 13.3 Laptop with stand, external keyboard and external mouse

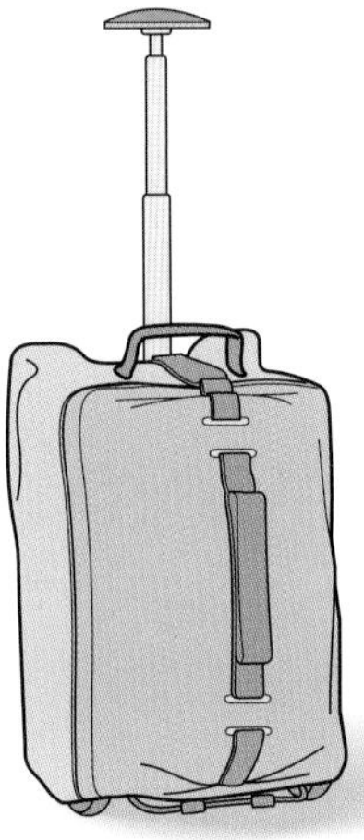

Figure 13.4 Laptop rucksack with wheels

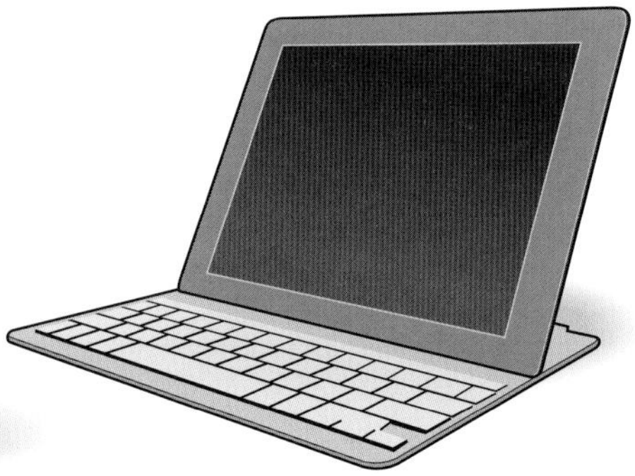

Figure 13.5 External keyboard for a tablet device

Figure 13.6 Pressure on the cervical spine when using a mobile device such as a tablet or mobile phone.
Source: Hansraj KK. *Surg Technol Int*. 2014;25:277–279

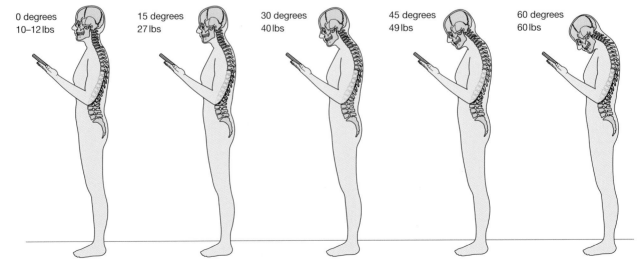

| 0 degrees 10–12 lbs | 15 degrees 27 lbs | 30 degrees 40 lbs | 45 degrees 49 lbs | 60 degrees 60 lbs |

There is a lot of clear guidance about sitting at a desk top computer (see Chapter 12). With the advent of laptops, tablets and smart phones, many of the recommendations are not able to be implemented without some creative thinking and the application of some ergonomic principles.

Laptops

The laptop allows mobile working and this means:

• There is no need to sit at a desk and you can work anywhere.

This means that you can have the laptop on your lap (as the name suggests) which means that it is too low and hence putting strain on your neck. Alternatively it can be used on tables in trains which are usually too high, putting strain on the neck and the lower back (see Chapter 4, Posture and back care).

The way to improve your posture when using a laptop is to create an environment that mimics that of a desk top computer. This requires three pieces of equipment:

1   A laptop stand. There are a number of these on the market and some can easily be transported with the laptop so that they can be used when travelling (Figure 13.1).

2   An external keyboard. Again there are many examples of these including flexible rubber ones that can be rolled up and make them easily portable (Figure 13.2).

3   A mouse that can be fitted into the USB socket.

An example of this set up can be seen in Figure 13.3.

• This is a piece of equipment that needs to be carried around.

Laptop bags are often carried over one shoulder; this means that the person carrying the laptop has their back, neck and shoulders out of alignment.

This can be addressed by using a laptop bag which is a rucksack and is then carried with both straps over the shoulders. The best solution is to have a rucksack that also has wheels. This allows the laptop to be both carried and also wheeled as necessary. An example of this is shown in Figure 13.4.

Tablets

There is an increasing use of this type of device which often causes the user to adopt poor postures, often for lengthy periods of time. There are external keyboards and stands for these devices, but effectively these convert the tablet to a conventional laptop. An example of this is shown in Figure 13.5. The key points are to:

• Use a stand as this changes your viewing angle.
• Change your posture regularly.
• Take a break every 15 minutes.
• If you are using your tablet without using the keyboard, use the device like a book and bring it up close to you, to avoid the 'vulture posture' with your neck.

Smart phones

All of the above issues with tablets apply to smart phones, but with a smaller screen and a greater likelihood of a poor posture that affects your neck and thoracic area of the spine. Minimising the time on the device and taking regular breaks will help reduce the risk of cumulative injury. Figure 13.6 shows the excessive pressure on the cervical spine when the phone is held low and not used held up to the face.

In general

Adopting a good posture when you are using these devices and taking regular breaks is the key. However, due to their portability it is easy to use them in places where good posture is difficult, such as on the sofa and in bed. In these locations it is easy to spend lengthy periods of time working, without being aware of poor posture.

14 Assessing the patient before standing from a chair

Figure 14.1 Ask the patient to raise their knee up against the side of your hand

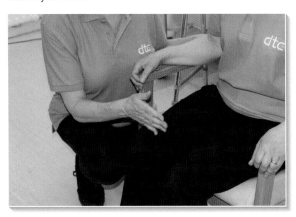

Figure 14.2 Ask the patient to straighten their leg by touching our hand with their toes

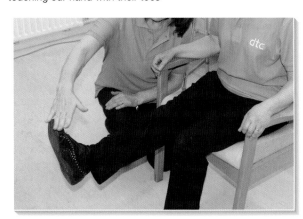

Figure 14.3 Make a bit of resistance with your hand as the patient brings their foot back to the floor

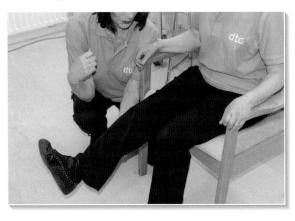

Figure 14.4 Ask the patient to push down on your hands

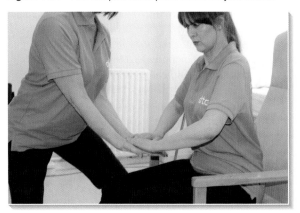

Figure 14.5 Ask the patient to move forward in the chair

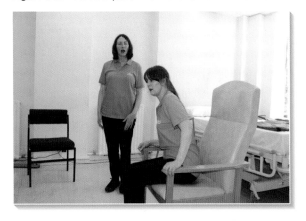

Figure 14.6 Check the patient's sitting balance by asking them to remove their hands from the arms of the chair

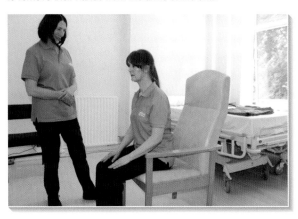

Moving and Handling Patients at a Glance. First Edition. Hamish MacGregor. © 2016 John Wiley & Sons, Ltd. Published 2016 by John Wiley & Sons, Ltd.

Purpose

To assess whether the patient can safely stand from the chair. The assessment will check if the patient has:

- Strength and movement in their legs and arms.
- Trunk control and sitting balance.
- The ability to understand and follow instructions relating to this handling task.

Prior to the assessment

1 Consult any handling plans relating to this patient. Check that they are clear, up-to-date and regularly reviewed.

2 If there is no written plan ask your colleagues if they have relevant information relating to this patient.

3 Communicate with the patient and tell them what you plan to do. Ensure that they understand and obtain their consent.

4 Ensure that the patient has suitable footwear before they attempt to stand, for example, flat enclosed shoes.

During the assessment

1 Get down to the side of the patient's chair. Be careful to ensure that you have a good posture.

2 Ask if you can put the edge of your hand on their knee and ask if they can lift their knee up against your hand (Figure 14.1). This will allow you to test if the patient has strength in their quadriceps. Do not use the flat of your hand as this can appear quite invasive to some patients and can compromise their dignity.

3 Ask the patient to straighten their leg and place your hand so that patient can aim for it (Figure 14.2). The patient needs to be able to fully straighten their leg.

4 As the patient brings their leg down, put your hand underneath the patient's calf and feel the resistance on the way down (Figure 14.3).

5 Move round to the other side of the chair and repeat the procedure. Note: If there are two handlers then it is important that only one does the assessment of both legs.

6 Stand in stable base in front of the patient and get them to push gently down on your hands. Check that the arm strength is equal (Figure 14.4). Note: Stand with your feet shoulder width apart, one foot in slightly in front of the other with flexed knees and your weight balanced between them. (A stable base is described fully in the key safe principles in Chapter 5.)

7 Ask the patient to shuffle forward in the chair, holding on to the arms of the chair (Figure 14.5).

8 If they cannot manage to move forward in the chair on their own. See Chapter 15, Moving a patient forwards in a chair.

9 Once the patient is forward in the chair ask the patient to put their hands on their knees. This will allow you to assess if they have any sitting balance. Patients may cover up poor balance by keeping hold of the arms of the chair (Figure 14.6).

10 During this task you will also be able to assess whether the patient has good cognition, as they will have had to follow instructions.

After the assessment

1 Check that the patient has no pain and/or discomfort.

2 Ensure that they are far enough forward in the chair to stand.

3 If the patient uses any walking aids, ensure that they are at hand, and the patient can reach them easily when preparing to stand up.

15 Moving a patient forwards in a chair

Figure 15.1 Move beside the patient, maintaining a good posture

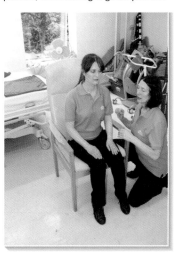

Figure 15.2 Encourage the patient to lean to the side with their weight off their opposite hip and thigh

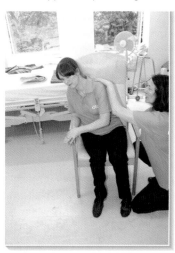

Figure 15.3 Ask the patient if you can place your hand on their hip and thigh

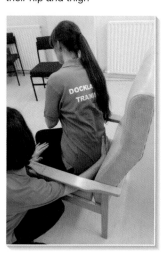

Figure 15.4 Gently move the patient's hip and thigh forward

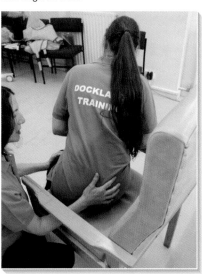

Figure 15.5 You can encourage the patient to move forward themselves by placing your hand in front of their knee and ask them to 'aim' for it

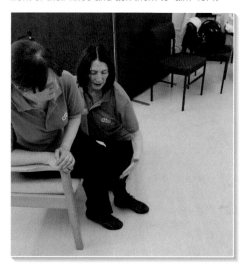

Figure 15.6 Repeat on the opposite side if necessary

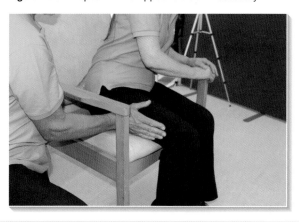

Moving and Handling Patients at a Glance. First Edition. Hamish MacGregor. © 2016 John Wiley & Sons, Ltd. Published 2016 by John Wiley & Sons, Ltd.

Purpose

To assist a patient to move forward in the chair who has difficulty doing so.

Prior to the handling task

1   Consult any handling plans relating to this patient and check that they are clear, up-to-date and regularly reviewed.

2   If there is no written plan, ask your colleagues if they have relevant information relating to this patient.

3   Communicate with the patient and tell them what you plan to do. Ensure that they understand and obtain their consent.

4   Make a final check that the patient cannot do this for themselves before continuing with the task.

During the task

1   Get down to the side of the patient's chair. Ensure that you have a good posture (Figure 15.1).

2   Ask the patient to lean over to the opposite side of the chair away from you. Place their hand nearest to you on the arm of the chair on the opposite side. This will allow the patient to take the weight off their hip nearest to you. At the same time ask the patient to keep their weight and head forward (Figure 15.2).

3   If the patient is anxious or fearful, it may be necessary to have another handler at the opposite side of the chair to reassure the patient.

4   Ask the patient if you can place your hand behind the patient's buttock and the flat of your other hand on the patient's thigh (Figure 15.3). Be very sensitive to the invasive nature of this and be aware that the patient may not find this acceptable, for example if the patient is female and you, as the handler, are male then it may be necessary to get a female handler to carry out this part of the task.

5   Gently move the patient's hip and thigh forward in a small controlled move (Figure 15.4). Remember the patient's hip and thigh must not be on the surface of the chair as they move their leg as the shearing forces could damage the skin.

6   Alternatively, if you place your other hand just in front, but not touching, the patient's knee this will give them something to aim for as they move their leg forward. This encourages the patient to fully participate in the manoeuvre (Figure 15.5).

7   Repeat on the opposite side if needed (Figure 15.6).

8   Often one small move is enough for a patient who has been sitting for a long time, as once they have made the initial move then the next one is easier. Always check this before moving to the other side of the chair and assisting the patients as we want to maximise the patient's independence.

After the task

1   Check that the patient has no pain and/or discomfort.

2   Ensure that they are far enough forward in the chair to stand.

3   If the patient uses any walking aids ensure that they are at hand and the patient can easily reach them when he/she is standing.

16 Standing a patient: with one handler

Figure 16.1 Place your hand on the patient's lower back

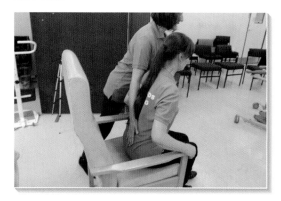

Figure 16.2 Alternatively, place your hand on the patient's iliac crest, if it does not involve too much stretching

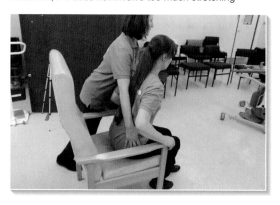

Figure 16.3 Place your other hand in front of the patient's shoulder

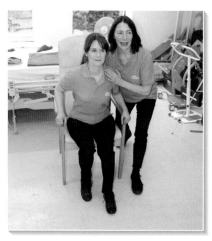

Figure 16.4 Giving clear instructions such as 'Ready, Steady, Stand', encourage the patient to stand up

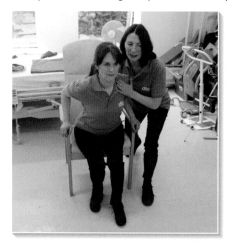

Figure 16.5 When the patient is standing, keep your hands in place until your patient is steady

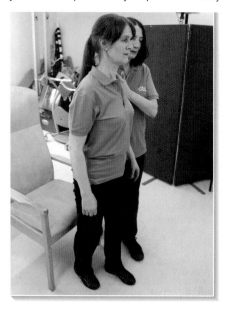

Figure 16.6 Offer the patient a palm to palm grip with your thumb tucked in

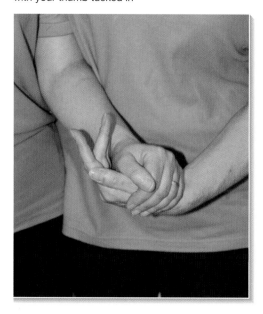

Moving and Handling Patients at a Glance. First Edition. Hamish MacGregor. © 2016 John Wiley & Sons, Ltd. Published 2016 by John Wiley & Sons, Ltd.

Purpose

To safely stand a patient from a chair whilst maintaining a good posture.

Prior to the handling task

1 Consult any handling plans relating to this patient and check that they are clear, up-to-date and regularly reviewed.

2 If there is no written plan, ask your colleagues if they have relevant information relating to this patient.

3 Ensure a suitable and sufficient assessment has been carried out beforehand. See Chapter 14, Assessing the patient before standing from a chair.

4 Ensure that the patient has suitable footwear before they attempt to stand, that is, flat enclosed shoes.

5 Communicate with the patient and tell them what you plan to do. Ensure that they understand and obtain their consent.

6 Make a final check that the patient cannot do this for themselves before continuing with the task.

7 Ensure that they are at the front of the chair. See Chapter 15, Moving a patient forwards in a chair.

During the task

1 Stand at the side of the patient's chair in a walk stance position with your feet in the direction you are facing with your inside leg back and outside leg in front.

2 Ask the patient to put one foot in front of the other. If the patient has a weakness on one side, check again if it is safe to stand them, and if so, ensure their strong leg is placed back and the weak leg is placed forward. You will need to stand on the weak side. If necessary get the help of another handler to stand on the opposite side.

3 Place your hand nearest the patient in the centre of their lower back below the waist line (Figure 16.1) or, if it does not involve too much stretching, put your hand on the opposite iliac crest (Figure 16.2).

4 Place your hand furthest away from the patient, in front of the patient's shoulder (Figure 16.3).

5 Using the clear verbal instructions of 'Ready, Steady, Stand', ask the patient to stand up, bringing their head forward with their nose coming over their toes and pushing with their arms on the side of the chair. *The patient should be leading the move with you guiding.* Do not rock the patient unless it has been identified in the risk assessment that this is necessary (Figure 16.4). Avoid using *1, 2, 3*, as the patient may be unsure if they move on the 3 or the imaginary 4. See Chapter 6, Controversial techniques. An exception to this may be with a patient who has stood successfully at home on '1, 2, 3', with carers but due to problems of cognition, such as dementia or learning disability, it may be difficult to learn new commands. In this case it is incumbent on the handlers to find out if the patient stands on 3 or the imaginary 4. This then needs to be documented in the patient's handling plan and communicated to the rest of the team.

6 When the patient has stood up, stay close by them, keeping your hand around their back and your hand on the shoulder until they are steady (Figure 16.5).

7 Offer them your hand that is on their shoulder in a palm to palm grip with thumbs tucked in (Figure 16.6).

8 If appropriate, hand the patient their walking frame or aid. If you are using a walking frame, ensure that it is in good condition and is the correct height for the patient. See Chapter 21, Tips for using walking frames, Do's and Don'ts, for more information.

After the task

1 Check that the patient is safe and comfortable.

2 Document if the patient experiences any dizziness, light-headedness or other symptoms that may put them at risk.

17 Standing a patient: with two handlers

Figure 17.1 Facing the same direction as the patient, cross your arms closest to the patient around the patient's back

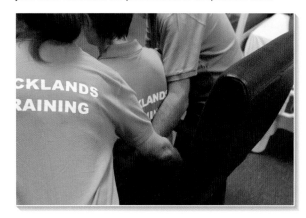

Figure 17.2 Your hands should be on the patient's iliac crest

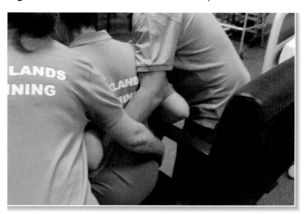

Figure 17.3 Place your other hand on the patient's shoulder

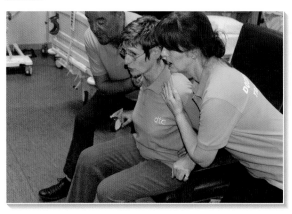

Figure 17.4 Giving clear instructions such as 'Ready, Steady, Stand', encourage the patient to stand up

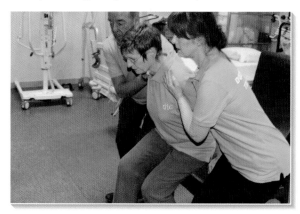

Figure 17.5 When the patient has stood, keep your hands in place until the patient is steady

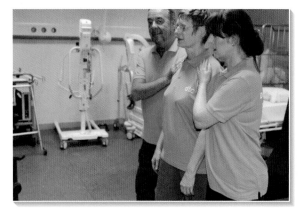

Figure 17.6 Offer the patient a palm to palm grip with your thumb tucked in

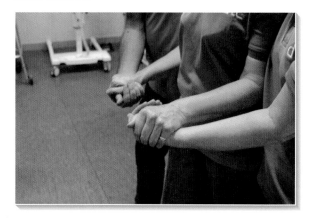

Moving and Handling Patients at a Glance. First Edition. Hamish MacGregor. © 2016 John Wiley & Sons, Ltd. Published 2016 by John Wiley & Sons, Ltd.

Purpose

To safely stand a patient from a chair whilst maintaining a good posture.

Prior to the handling task

1 Consult any handling plans relating to this patient and check that they are clear, up-to-date and regularly reviewed.

2 If there is no written plan, ask your colleagues if they have relevant information relating to this patient.

3 Ensure a suitable and sufficient assessment has been carried out beforehand. This will include an up-to-date Falls Assessment if appropriate.

4 Ensure that the patient has suitable footwear before they attempt to stand, that is, flat enclosed shoes.

5 Communicate with the patient and tell them what you plan to do. Ensure that they understand and obtain their consent.

6 Refer to Chapter 14, Assessing the patient before standing from a chair.

7 Ensure that they are at the front of the chair. See Chapter 15, Moving a patient forwards in a chair.

8 **Please note.** The reason for using this technique may not be to do with the patient's abilities but environmental factors such as the chair being too low. The pictures opposite show the patient in a low chair and this has necessitated using two handlers.

During the task

1 Stand at either side of the patient's chair in a walk stance position with your feet in the direction you are facing. See Chapter 16, Standing a patient from a chair with one handler, for more information on this. Both handlers' arms need to be crossed around the patient's back (Figures 17.1 and 17.2).

2 Ask the patient to put one foot in front of the other. If the patient has a weakness on one side, check again if it is safe to stand them, if so, ensure their strong leg is placed back and the weak leg is placed forward.

3 With your arms cupped on the patient's shoulders prepare to move the patient (Figure 17.3).

4 Using the clear verbal instructions of 'Ready, Steady, Stand,' ask the patient to stand up, bringing their head forward with their nose coming over their toes and pushing with their arms on the side of the chair. *The patient should be leading the move with you guiding.*

- Do not rock the patient unless it has been identified in the risk assessment that this is necessary (Figure 17.4).
- Avoid using *1, 2, 3*, as the patient may be unsure if they move on the 3 or the imaginary 4.
- See Chapter 6, Controversial techniques, for more information on this.
- An exception to this is may be with a patient who has stood successfully at home on 1, 2, 3, with carers, but due to problems of cognition, such as dementia or learning disability, it may be difficult to learn new commands. In this case it is incumbent on the handlers to find out if the patient stands on 3 or the imaginary 4. This then needs to be documented in the patient's handling plan and communicated to the rest of the team.

5 When the patient has stood up, stay close by them, keeping your hands around their back and your hand on their shoulder until they are steady (Figure 17.5).

6 Offer them your hand that is on their shoulder in a palm to palm grip with thumbs tucked in (Figure 17.6).

7 If appropriate, hand the patient their walking frame or aid. If you are using a walking frame ensure that it is in good condition and is the correct height for the patient. See Chapter 21, Tips for using walking frames, and further information.

After the task

1 Check that the patient is safe and comfortable.

2 Document if the patient experiences any dizziness, lightheadedness or other symptoms that may put them at risk.

(18) Seating a patient

Figure 18.1 Ensure the patient can see the chair as you approach it

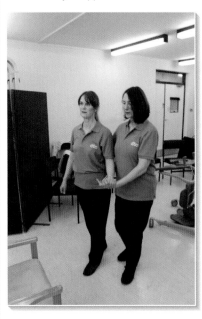

Figure 18.2 Ensure that you are at the opposite side of the patient, furthest from the chair

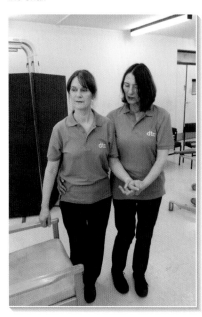

Figure 18.3 Ensure the patient can feel the back of the chair with their legs

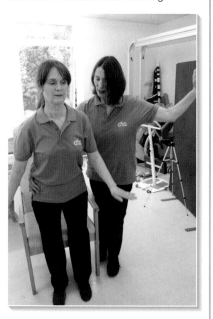

Figure 18.4 Ask the patient to feel for the arms of the chair

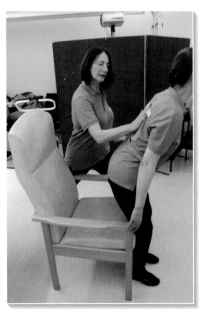

Figure 18.5 As the patient sits down, place your hand between their shoulder blades

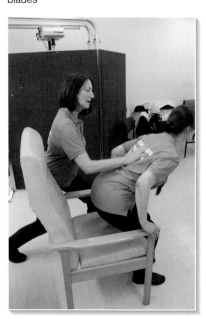

Figure 18.6 Remove your hand as the patient sits down

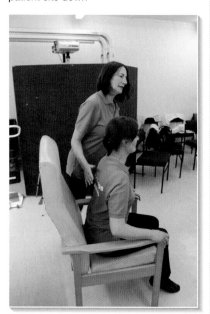

Moving and Handling Patients at a Glance. First Edition. Hamish MacGregor. © 2016 John Wiley & Sons, Ltd. Published 2016 by John Wiley & Sons, Ltd.

Purpose

To sit a patient down safely in a chair while maintaining a good posture.

Prior to the handling task

1   As you will probably have been walking the patient prior to this, ensure that you are clear about how to walk a patient safely. See Chapter 20, Walking with handler(s).

2   Consult any handling plans relating to this patient and check that they are clear, up-to-date and regularly reviewed.

3   If there is no written plan, ask your colleagues if they have relevant information relating to this patient.

4   Communicate with the patient and tell them what you plan to do. Ensure that they understand and obtain their consent.

During the task

1   As you are walking a patient to the chair, ensure that they can see the chair and you, as the handler, are not blocking the chair (Figures 18.1 and 18.2). This is very important, because if you block the chair, the patient has to walk backwards into the chair and this could cause dizziness or uncertainty as to its exact location.

2   As the patient backs into the chair, ensure that they can feel the chair at back of their knees (Figure 18.3). If the patient cannot feel the back of the chair with their legs they cannot be sure that the chair is there, and this may cause them to have feelings of uncertainty.

3   Ask the patient to reach for the arms of the chair, one hand at a time. Ask the patient to bring their head forward and aim for the back of the chair (Figure 18.4). The use of clear verbal instructions such as 'Ready, Steady, Sit', are important to the patient as this acts as another prompt for them to sit.

4   Ensure that you are in a walk stance position at the side of the chair, with your inside leg back, and move your hand into the centre of the patient's back between the shoulder blades. This will encourage the patient to bring their head forward and get their hips to the back of the chair (Figure 18.5).

5   Remove your hand as the patient reaches the back of the chair. This will allow the patient to get fully to the back of the chair (Figure 18.6).

After the task

1   Check that the patient is far enough back in the chair and that they are safe and comfortable.

2   Document any findings in the handling plan as necessary.

19 Moving a patient back in a chair

Figure 19.1 Place the flat of your hand nearest the patient on their thigh

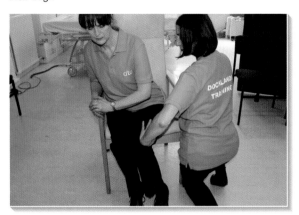

Figure 19.2 Place your other hand on their hip

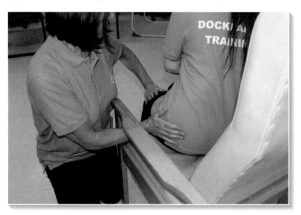

Figure 19.3 Move the patient's hip and thigh back in a small controlled movement

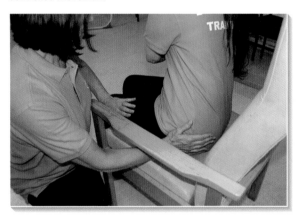

Figure 19.4 Move to the opposite side of the patient

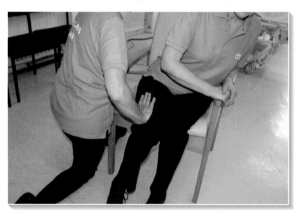

Figure 19.5 Repeat as in Figures 19.1, 19.2 and 19.3

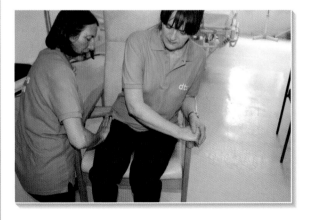

Figure 19.6 Ensure the patient is fully back in the chair

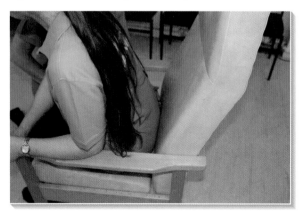

Moving and Handling Patients at a Glance. First Edition. Hamish MacGregor. © 2016 John Wiley & Sons, Ltd. Published 2016 by John Wiley & Sons, Ltd.

Purpose

To assist a patient to move back in the chair who has difficulty doing so.

Prior to the handling task

1   Consult any handling plans relating to this patient and check that they are clear, up-to-date and regularly reviewed.

2   If there is no written plan, ask your colleagues if they have relevant information relating to this patient.

3   Communicate with the patient and tell them what you plan to do. Ensure that they understand and obtain their consent.

4   Make a final check that the patient cannot do this for themselves before continuing with the task.

5   If the patient was sat fully back in the chair when they first sat down, this task will not be necessary. See Chapter 18, Seating a patient.

6   For some patients it may be easier to ask them, or assist them, to stand again.

During the task

1   Get down to the side of the patient's chair. Ensure you have good posture.

2   Ask the patient to lean over to the opposite side of the chair away from you. Place their hand nearest to you on the arm of the chair on the opposite side. This will allow the patient to take the weight off their hip nearest to you. At the same time ask the patient to keep their weight and head forward. This is the reverse of the procedure of moving a patient forwards in the chair. See Chapter 15 for more details if necessary.

3   Ask the patient if you can place your hand behind the patient's buttock and the flat of your other hand on the patient's thigh (Figure 19.1). Be very sensitive to the invasive nature of this and be aware that the patient may not find this acceptable, for example, if the patient is female and you, as the handler, are male then it may be necessary to ask a female handler to carry out this part of the task.

4   Your other hand should be behind the patient's hip (Figure 19.2).

5   Gently move the patient's hip and thigh back in a small controlled move (Figure 19.3). Remember, the patient's hip and thigh must be slightly raised and not be on the surface of the chair, as the shearing forces could damage the skin.

6   Move to the opposite side of the chair and repeat the process (Figures 19.4 and 19.5).

7   Ensure the patient has reached the back of the chair with their feet flat on the floor (Figure 19.6).

After the task

1   Check that the patient has no pain and/or discomfort.

2   If the patient is starting to slip forward in the chair an additional assessment needs to take place looking at:

- Height of chair.
- Depth of seat.
- Need for a footstool?
- Is a specialist seat necessary to give the patient the correct level of support?

If any of the above issues need to be addressed you may have to enlist the help of another health or social care professional, such as an occupational therapist.

20 Walking with handler(s)

Figure 20.1   Cross your arms around the patient's back

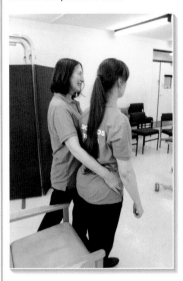

Figure 20.2   Offer the patient your upturned hand

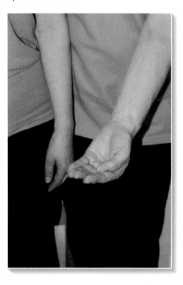

Figure 20.3   Palm grip with thumbs tucked in

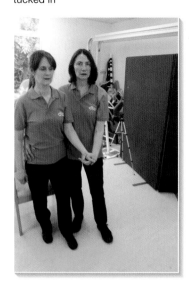

Figure 20.4   Move forward together

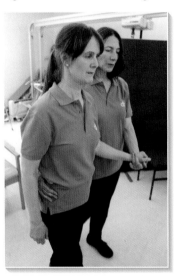

Figure 20.5   Do not allow the patient to look at the floor

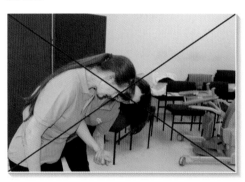

Figure 20.6   Offer the patient a walking frame if needed once they are standing

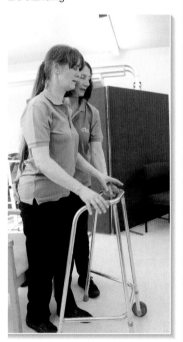

Figure 20.8   If there are two handlers, arms are crossed around the patient's back

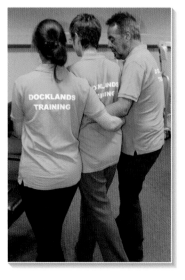

Figure 20.7   If there are two handlers, both have a palm to palm grip

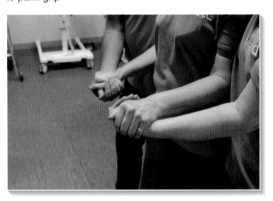

Moving and Handling Patients at a Glance. First Edition. Hamish MacGregor. © 2016 John Wiley & Sons, Ltd. Published 2016 by John Wiley & Sons, Ltd.

Purpose

To walk a patient safely while maintaining a good posture.

Prior to the handling task

1   Consult any handling plans relating to this patient and check that they are clear, up-to-date and regularly reviewed.

2   If there is no written plan, ask your colleagues if they have relevant information relating to this patient.

3   Ensure a suitable and sufficient assessment has been carried out beforehand.

4   Ensure that the patient has suitable footwear before they attempt to walk, that is, flat enclosed shoes.

5   Communicate with the patient and tell them what you plan to do. Ensure that they understand and obtain their consent.

6   Refer to Chapter 14, Assessing the patient before standing from a chair, if you need to stand the patient prior to this task.

7   Refer to Chapter 16, Standing a patient, as this may have been carried out prior to this procedure.

During the task

1   Stand at the side of the patient in a walk stance position with your feet facing forward. Your arm closest to the patient needs to be crossed around the patient's back (Figure 20.1).

2   When the patient is ready offer them your hand, palm up with your thumb tucked in, then allow the patient to place their palm on your palm (Figures 20.2 and 20.3).

3   When the patient is ready, all walk forward together, giving the patient enough space to walk normally by moving their hips (Figure 20.4).

• Do try and keep your hand at the level of a walking stick that the patient may use.

• Do beware of allowing your hand and the patient's hand to rise up as this will give less control.

• Do not allow the patient to put their weight through your hand. If this happens politely ask the patient to stop. Asking them to keep their head up and look ahead often prevents the patient from doing this.

4   Encourage the patient to keep their head up and look ahead.

• Do not allow the patient to look down at the floor (Figure 20.5). Simple verbal instructions such as 'Head up' and 'Stand up straight' can be helpful.

5   If using a walking frame, walk at the side of the patient with one hand on their back and one hand on the frame (Figure 20.6). See Chapter 21, Tips for using walking frames, for further information.

6   If your assessment indicates, have a person walking behind with a wheelchair.

7   Please refer to Chapter 18, Seating a patient, if appropriate.

8   When the patient needs more assistance, this technique may require two handlers. All of the above applies, but ensure both hands are in a palm to palm grip with the patient (Figure 20.7) and the handlers' hands are crossed around the patient's back (Figure 20.8). This should give the patient more reassurance and confidence when they are being walked.

After the task

1   Check that the patient is safe and comfortable.

2   Document if the patient experiences any dizziness, light-headedness or other symptoms that may put them at risk.

21 Tips for using walking frames

Figure 21.1 Ensure the patient is fully stood up before they take their frame

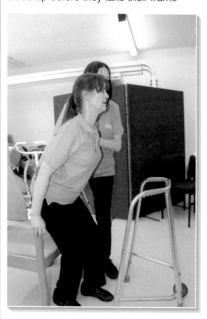

Figure 21.2 Hand the patient the frame if they are unable to stand into it

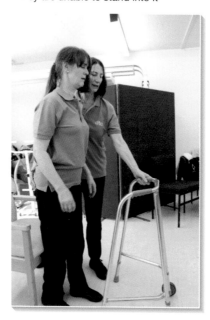

Figure 21.3 DO NOT allow the patient to stand using the frame

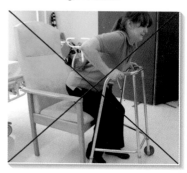

Figure 21.4 DO NOT lean on the side of the frame

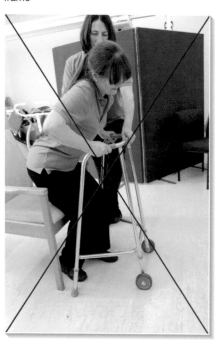

Figure 21.5 DO NOT lean on the front of the frame

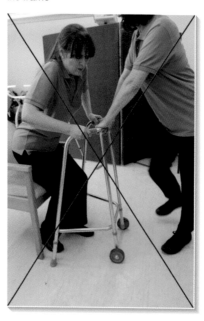

Figure 21.6 DO NOT put your foot on the frame

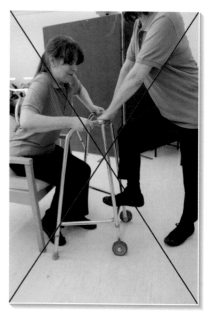

Moving and Handling Patients at a Glance. First Edition. Hamish MacGregor. © 2016 John Wiley & Sons, Ltd. Published 2016 by John Wiley & Sons, Ltd.

Purpose

To identify the correct use of the walking frame and the hazards associated with incorrect use.

A walking frame is a stable walking device that allows the patient to walk within the area of support provided by the walking frame's base. The walking frame is usually lifted forward by the patient and the patient steps forward into the frame one foot at a time. Some frames have wheels (often called rollators) and these are pushed forward by the patient rather than lifted.

DO

1 Ensure the frame is the correct size for the patient. If in doubt check with the physiotherapist, occupational therapist or other relevant professional.

2 Ensure that the patient knows how to use the frame and is confident to walk with it.

3 Stand the patient up as described in Chapter 16, Standing a patient with one handler; or Chapter 17, Standing a patient with two handlers. The frame should be in front of the patient, but not close enough to inhibit them from standing correctly (Figure 21.1).

4 Once the patient has stood up, hand them the walking frame if they are unable to step towards it (Figure 21.2).

5 Use two people to stand the person if the assessment indicates.

6 Have a person walking behind with a wheelchair if the patient is anxious, easily fatigued or has a history of falls.

DON'T

1 Allow the patient to use the walking frame as a standing aid (Figure 21.3). This does not allow the patient to use natural body movement and the frame is unstable and could topple over.

2 Lean on the frame from the side (Figure 21.4) or from the front (Figure 21.5). The patient may ask you to do this, but it does not allow the patient to use natural body movement, so puts them at risk. This assessment is particularly important if they are going home from hospital. If there is no-one at home to stabilise the frame, they might not be able to get up from the chair. If this is an ongoing problem an occupational therapy assessment might be needed to assess for a riser recliner chair.

3 Put your foot on the frame (Figure 21.6). All of the above applies, but additionally this will weaken the frame as this part of the frame is not designed to be stood upon. If it breaks you could injure yourself or the patient.

22 Assisting a patient off the floor: verbal

Figure 22.1 Ask the patient to turn on their side, knees bent and with the palm of their hand on the floor

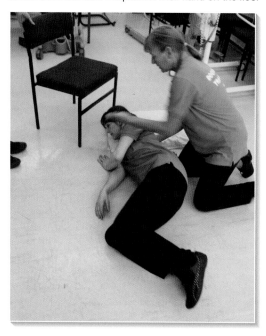

Figure 22.2 Ask the patient to push up with their hand and then rest on their elbow

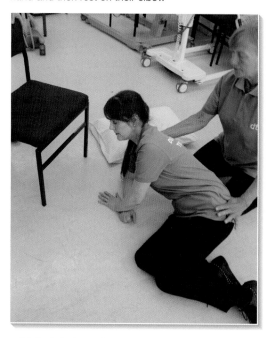

Figure 22.3 Ask the patient to move onto their knees

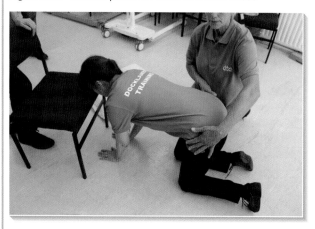

Figure 22.4 Ask the patient to put their arms on the first chair

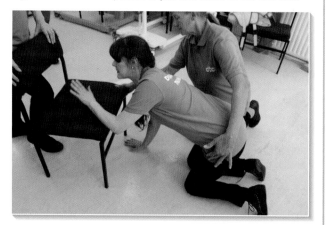

Figure 22.5 Ask the patient to push up onto one foot

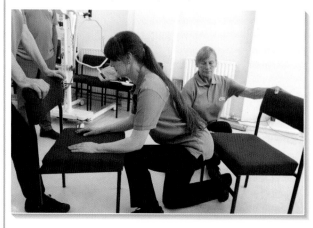

Figure 22.6 Ask the patient to sit back onto the second chair

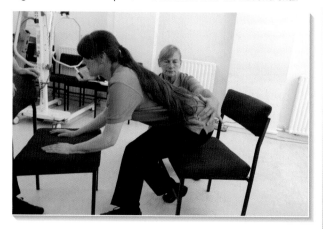

Moving and Handling Patients at a Glance. First Edition. Hamish MacGregor. © 2016 John Wiley & Sons, Ltd. Published 2016 by John Wiley & Sons, Ltd.

Purpose

To assist a patient from the floor using verbal commands.

Prior to the handling task

1 Consult any handling plans relating to this patient and check that they are clear, up-to-date and regularly reviewed.

2 If there is no written plan, ask your colleagues if they have relevant information relating to this patient.

3 Check that the patient is not injured. Ask them if they have any pain. Ascertain how they fell and the circumstances surrounding the fall.

4 Check the patient's blood pressure, neurological observations or any other tests deemed necessary at the time.

5 Ensure that the patient has suitable footwear before they attempt to walk, such as flat enclosed shoes.

6 Communicate with the patient and tell them what you plan to do. Ensure that they understand and obtain their consent.

During the task

1 Get down to the patient's level on the floor; be aware of your posture as you do this. The second handler should place two chairs nearby.

2 Ask the patient to turn on their side with their legs bent at the knees and their upper arm, palm down on the floor (Figure 22.1).

3 When the patient is ready, ask them to push up with the hand on the floor and get them to rest on the elbow of their other arm. This is called three-point sitting (Figure 22.2). The patient may need to have a rest here before continuing to the next stage.

4 When the patient is ready, ask them to move onto their knees (four-point sitting) (Figure 22.3). It is often useful to place your hands on either side of the patient's hip to give reassurance. Ensure that you have asked permission first. The patient may need to have a rest here before continuing to the next stage.

5 The second handler places one chair in front of the patient so that the patient can put their arms on the chair. When the patient is ready, ask them to push up onto one foot while pushing on the chair with their arms for stability (Figure 22.4).

6 Then ask the patient to push up onto their other foot while the first handler places the second chair behind them (Figure 22.5).

7 When the patient can feel the back of the second chair behind their knees they can then sit down (Figure 22.6).

8 If at any point the patient cannot manage this, stop and use an alternative method such as a hoist.

9 Keep your instructions simple and short. It may be necessary to get down on the floor with the patient and mirror what you want them to do. This will mean you being directly in front of them and showing the patient all the steps mentioned above by demonstrating exactly what you want them to do.

10 This task takes time and at no stage should the patient be hurried.

11 Remember the patient may be fearful and anxious and will require constant reassurance.

After the task

1 Check that the patient is safe and comfortable.

2 Document if the patient experiences any dizziness, light-headedness or other symptoms that may put them at risk.

3 Complete an incident report form in line with your organisation's policies.

4 Revise the patient's falls risk assessment profile. Communicate this to all members of the care team.

23 Sitting a patient using an electric profiling bed

Figure 23.1 Auto profile button (yellow)

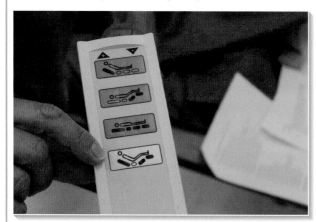

Figure 23.2 Knee break button first, then back rest button second

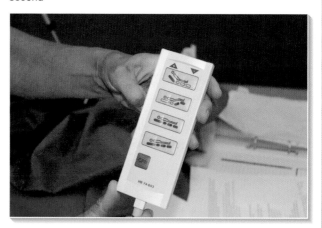

Figure 23.3 Bring back rest up, checking the patient's comfort level

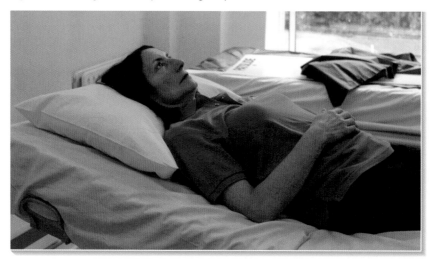

Figure 23.4 Using a small roller, slide sheet behind the patient's back

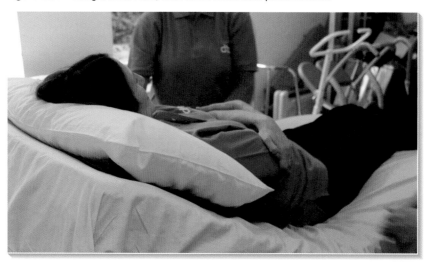

Moving and Handling Patients at a Glance. First Edition. Hamish MacGregor. © 2016 John Wiley & Sons, Ltd. Published 2016 by John Wiley & Sons, Ltd.

Purpose

To sit a patient up in bed who is unable to carry out the task themselves.

Prior to the handling task

1   Consult any handling plans relating to this patient and check that they are clear, up-to-date and regularly reviewed.

2   If there is no written plan, ask your colleagues if they have relevant information relating to this patient.

3   Communicate with the patient and tell them what you plan to do. Ensure that they understand and obtain their consent.

4   Make a final check that the patient cannot do this for themselves before continuing with the task.

5   The handlers must familiarise themselves with the bed controls. All makes of bed are different. Refer to the manufacturer's instructions if in any doubt.

6   Ensure that the bed is at the correct height, that is, at waist height of the shorter handler.

During the task

1   If the bed has an 'auto-profile function' where the knee break comes up slightly before the back rest, use it unless the risk assessment identifies a reason to do otherwise. See the yellow button (Figure 23.1). Once the patient is in a semi-seated position, then bring the backrest and knee break up independently to maximise the patient's comfort. Move the bed slowly, always checking with the patient that they are comfortable with the move. If appropriate, allow the patient to use the controls themselves.

2   If there is no 'auto-profile function' bring up the knee break, second button down (Figure 23.2). This may only need to be a small movement; check with the patient what is comfortable for them. Then bring up the back rest, top button (Figure 23.2). Again, if appropriate, allow the patient to use the controls themselves.

3   Both the above actions prevent the patient from sliding down the bed when the back rest is raised.

4   Slowly bring up the back rest, always checking the patient's level of comfort (Figure 23.3).

5   If the patient feels that the raising of the back rest is pulling on their back and shoulders, get them to bring their shoulders forward one at a time as the back rest is raised. This will reduce the pressure in this area.

6   If the patient is unable to do this, insert a small roller slide sheet under the patient's shoulders down to their lower back before raising the back rest (Figure 23.4).

7   For full information on inserting a roller slide sheet under the patient from the shoulders down see Chapter 35, Inserting a roller slide sheet under a patient: unravelling technique. Do note that it is a small slide sheet that is used, as it only needs to come down as far as the patient's lower back.

8   If the patient cannot sit forward, the slide sheet can be removed as described in Chapter 36, Moving a semi-independent patient up the bed on a roller slide sheet ('During the task', sections 4–6).

After the task

1   Check that the patient has no pain and/or discomfort.

2   Raise the bed rails if indicated in the handling plan ensuring there has been an up-to-date bed rails assessment form completed.

3   Raise the bed to the correct height for the patient.

Important: **The controls shown here are for one model of bed. All beds are different; ensure you familiarise yourself with a bed before you use it.**

24 Sitting a patient using a non-profiling bed

Figure 24.1 Ask the patient to bend their knees

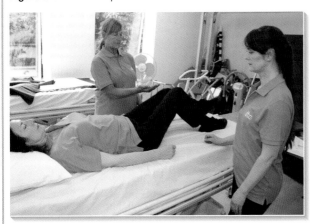

Figure 24.2 The patient and handler hold each other's elbows

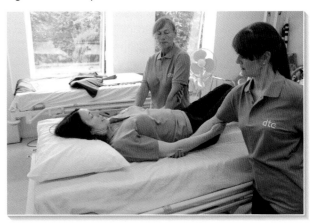

Figure 24.3 The handler's outer hand is placed on the bed and the patient's chin to their chest

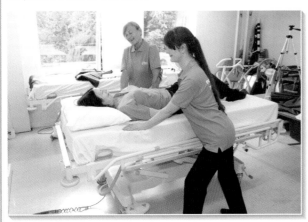

Figure 24.4 Adopting a walk stance position, the handlers transfer their weight back from their front leg to their back leg

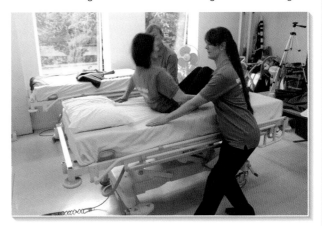

Figure 24.5 One handler crosses their arm over the patient's back

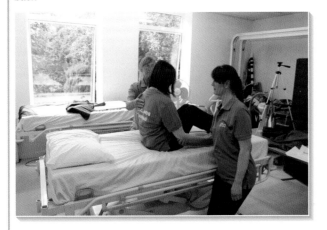

Figure 24.6 The same handler then places their other hand on the bed to stabilise the patient

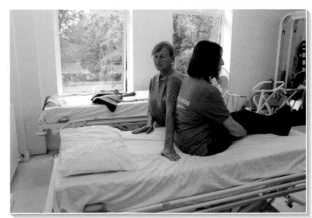

Moving and Handling Patients at a Glance. First Edition. Hamish MacGregor. © 2016 John Wiley & Sons, Ltd. Published 2016 by John Wiley & Sons, Ltd.

Purpose

To sit a patient up on the bed who is unable to carry out the task themselves.

This should never be a routine handling task and should only be used where the profiling bed has broken or the patient is awaiting for a more appropriate bed.

Prior to the handling task

1 Consult any handling plans relating to this patient and check that they are clear, up-to-date and regularly reviewed.

2 If there is no written plan, ask your colleagues if they have relevant information relating to this patient.

3 The patient must be able to hold the handler's elbows and have strength in their arms. Conditions such as arthritis may not be suitable for this manoeuvre.

4 Communicate with the patient and tell them what you plan to do. Ensure that they understand and obtain their consent.

5 Make a final check that the patient cannot do this for themselves before continuing with the task.

6 Ensure that the bed is at the correct height, that is, at waist height of the shorter handler.

During the task

1 Encourage the patient to bend their knees (Figure 24.1).

2 The handlers position themselves at either side of the bed. They must be close to the bed and in a walk stance position. The handler holds the patient's elbow and the patient holds the handler's elbow. THE PATIENT MUST HAVE THE ABILITY TO DO THIS. See point 3 in the previous section (Figure 24.2).

3 Both the handlers place their outer hand on the bed and encourage the patient to put their chin on their chest (Figure 24.3).

4 Both handlers adopt a walk stance position with their inside leg back and their outer leg forward. Using commands such as 'Ready, Steady, Sit' (or other clear commands agreed with the patient), both handlers transfer their weight back from their front leg to their back leg. The patient must maximise their cooperation at this time (Figure 24.4). If at any time during this manoeuvre it becomes too difficult for the patient or the handlers, you must stop, gently allow the patient to lie back down on the bed and look at an alternative method of carrying out this manoeuvre.

5 Once the patient has sat up (Figure 24.5), one of the handlers crosses their arm across the patient's back in order to stabilise them (Figure 24.6). This handler must be aware of their posture and have a broad base of support with flexed knees and ensure that their lower back is not twisted.

6 The second handler must immediately place pillows, a wedge or other support behind the patient's back. If it is an older bed, such as a King's Fund bed with a back rest that pulls out, it will be the second handler's role to pull out the back rest and arrange the pillows.

After the task

1 Check that the patient has no pain and/or discomfort.

2 Raise the bed rails if indicated in the handling plan, ensuring there has been an up-to-date bed rails assessment form completed.

3 Raise the bed to the correct height for the patient.

25 Sitting a patient onto the side of an electric profiling bed

Figure 25.1 Ask the patient to turn on their side, with their knees bent and with their upper hand on the bed

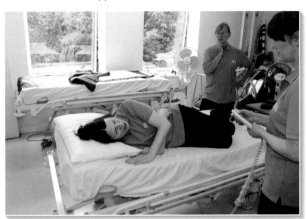

Figure 25.2 The head of the bed is raised to a maximum of 45 degrees

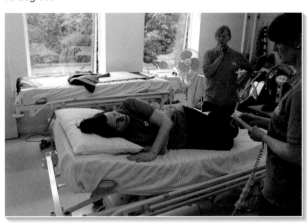

Figure 25.3 Ask the patient to swing their legs off the bed and push with their hand

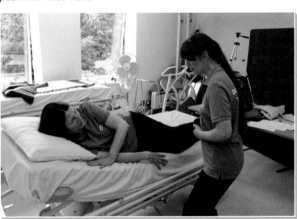

Figure 25.4 Encourage the patient to push themselves up until they are on the edge of the bed

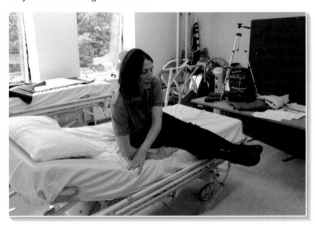

Figure 25.5 Ask the patient to move from hip to hip until they are on the edge of the bed

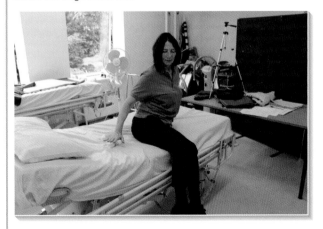

Figure 25.6 Ensure the bed is at a height such that the patient can place their feet on the floor

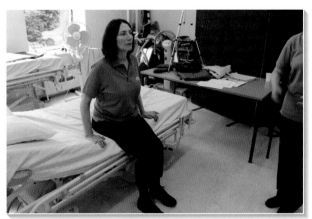

Moving and Handling Patients at a Glance. First Edition. Hamish MacGregor. © 2016 John Wiley & Sons, Ltd. Published 2016 by John Wiley & Sons, Ltd.

Purpose

To sit a patient up onto the side of the bed who is able to carry out the task themselves.

Prior to the handling task

1   Consult any handling plans relating to this patient and check that they are clear, up-to-date and regularly reviewed.

2   If there is no written plan, ask your colleagues if they have relevant information relating to this patient.

3   Communicate with the patient and tell them what you plan to do. Ensure that they understand and obtain their consent.

4   Make a final check that the patient cannot do this for themselves before continuing with the task.

5   The handler must familiarise themself with the bed controls. All makes of bed are different. Refer to the manufacturer's instructions if in any doubt.

6   Ensure that the bed is at the correct height, that is, that when the patient sits at the edge of the bed their feet reach the floor.

7   If the patient is short in stature and has difficulty placing their feet on the floor, check whether there is a facility on the bed that allows the bed to go down lower. This is quite common on more modern beds.

During the task

1   Ask the patient to turn onto their side with both knees bent and the hand of the upper arm flat on the bed. It is vital that the shoulder of the upper arm is kept forward (Figure 25.1). If this shoulder is allowed to move back the patient will not be able to get out of bed.

2   Bring the head of the bed up if the patient needs some assistance. The head of the bed should not be brought up to more than 45 degrees. Anything more than 45 degrees will mean that the side flexor muscles of the trunk will become shortened and this will make it harder work for the patient to get out of bed (Figure 25.2).

3   Ask the patient to swing their legs off the bed and push with the hand that is on the bed (Figure 25.3).

4   The patient continues to push themselves up until they have reached an upright position at the edge of the bed (Figure 25.4).

5   The patient moves from one hip to the other in order to reach the edge of the bed (Figure 25.5).

6   This is repeated until the patient has reached the edge of the bed and they have their feet flat on the floor (Figure 25.6).

7   In points 3 to 6 above, it may be necessary to be close to the patient to give them confidence and encouragement. If this is so, ensure that you adopt a good posture and avoid stooping.

8   If the patient requires a more hands on approach read Chapter 26, Sitting a patient onto the side of a non-profiling bed.

After the task

1   Check that the patient has no pain and/or discomfort.

2   Check that the patient is safe and is stable sitting on the edge of the bed.

26 Sitting a patient onto the side of a non-profiling bed

Figure 26.1 Ask the patient to turn onto their side, knees bent and with their upper hand on the bed

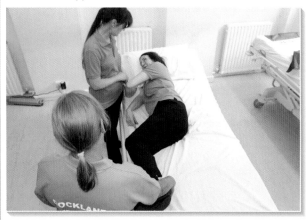

Figure 26.2 Place one hand on the patient's iliac crest and the other on their shoulder

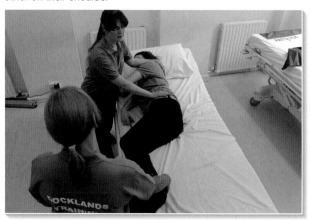

Figure 26.3 Encourage the patient to move their legs off the bed

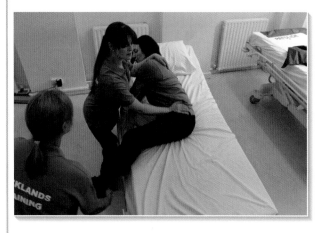

Figure 26.4 Once upright, encourage the patient to stabilise themselves

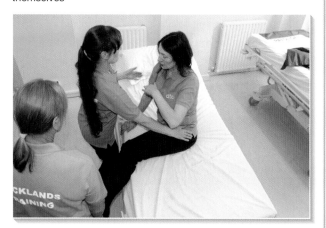

Figure 26.5 Ask the patient to move from hip to hip until they are at the edge of the bed

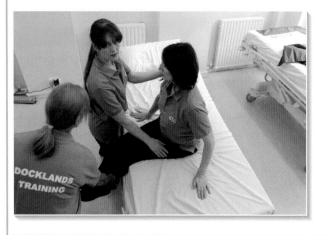

Figure 26.6 Ensure the patient's feet are flat on the floor

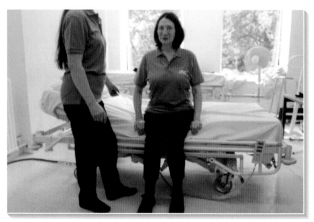

Moving and Handling Patients at a Glance. First Edition. Hamish MacGregor. © 2016 John Wiley & Sons, Ltd. Published 2016 by John Wiley & Sons, Ltd.

Purpose

To sit a patient up onto the side of the bed who is able to carry out the task themselves with guidance and/or minimal assistance.

Prior to the handling task

1 Consult any handling plans relating to this patient and check that they are clear, up-to-date and regularly reviewed.

2 If there is no written plan, ask your colleagues if they have relevant information relating to this patient.

3 Communicate with the patient and tell them what you plan to do. Ensure that they understand and obtain their consent.

4 Make a final check that the patient cannot do this for themselves before continuing with the task.

5 Ensure that the bed is at the correct height, that is, that when the patient sits at the edge of the bed their feet reach the floor.

During the task

1 Ask the patient to turn onto their side with both knees bent and the hand of the upper arm flat on the bed. It is vital that the shoulder of the upper arm is kept forward (Figure 26.1). If this shoulder is allowed to move back the patient will not be able to get out of bed.

2 Ask the patient to put their legs at the edge of the bed. Their knees should be in line with the edge of the mattress. Place one hand on the patient's iliac crest. The other hand should keep the patient's shoulder forward (Figure 26.2). A second handler can, if necessary, guide the patient's legs towards the edge of the bed.

3 Encourage the patient to drop their legs over the edge of the bed. Keep the patient's shoulder forward. Ensure that you have a broad base of support with your spine in line. Be careful not to stoop (Figure 26.3). A second handler can guide the patient's legs to the floor. This handler must bend at the hips and knees to avoid excessive stooping.

4 Once the patient is in an upright position encourage them to stabilise themselves, placing their hands flat on the bed (Figure 26.4).

5 Encourage the patient to move from hip to hip to move themselves to the edge of the bed (Figure 26.5).

6 Keep encouraging them to move themselves forward until their feet are flat on the floor (Figure 26.6).

7 It is important to assess how well the patient manages this task, if this is leading on to standing them up from the edge of the bed. See Chapter 28, Standing a patient up from the bed edge, and Chapter 29, Standing a patient up from the bed edge using a profiling bed (minimal assistance). This assessment may indicate the amount of assistance necessary or whether equipment may be needed.

After the task

1 Check that the patient has no pain and/or discomfort.

2 Check that the patient is safe and is stable sitting on the edge of the bed.

27 Lying down a patient from the bed edge

Figure 27.1 Ask the patient to put their right forearm on the bed

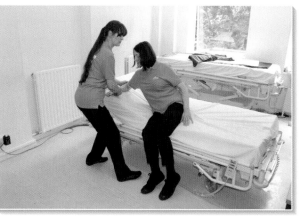

Figure 27.2 Ask the patient to lift one leg onto the bed. Ensure that their left shoulder is forward

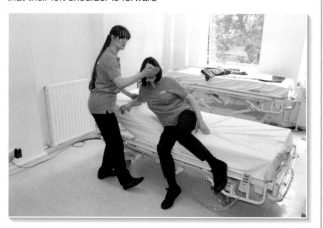

Figure 27.3 Ask the patient to lift their other leg onto the bed

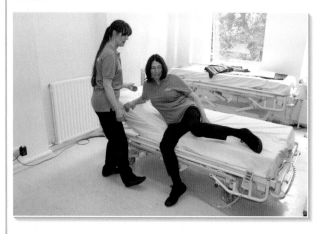

Figure 27.4 Once both legs are on the bed, the patient can swivel around

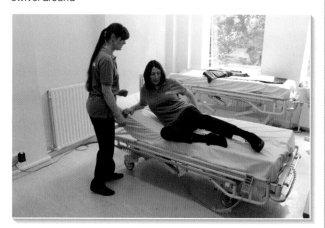

Figure 27.5 (a, b) Continue with small movements until the patient is comfortable on the bed

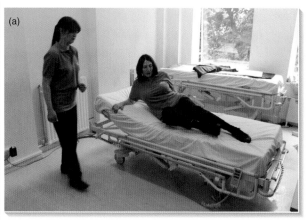

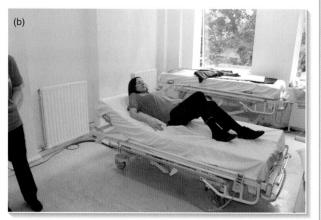

Moving and Handling Patients at a Glance. First Edition. Hamish MacGregor. © 2016 John Wiley & Sons, Ltd. Published 2016 by John Wiley & Sons, Ltd.

Purpose

To assist a patient into bed from the sitting on the edge of the bed.

Prior to the handling task

1   Consult any handling plans relating to this patient and check that they are clear, up-to-date and regularly reviewed.

2   If there is no written plan, ask your colleagues if they have relevant information relating to this patient.

3   Communicate with the patient and tell them what you plan to do. Ensure that they understand and obtain their consent.

4   Make a final check that the patient cannot do this for themselves before continuing with the task.

5   Ensure that the bed is at the correct height, that is, that when the patient sits at the edge of the bed their feet reach the floor.

During the task

Please note that the instruction here for right and left apply to these pictures. If the patient were getting into bed from the opposite side then right and left would be reversed.

1   Ask the patient to sit on the edge of the bed, ensuring that they are far enough up the bed and that they are in the correct position in the bed when they bring their legs onto the bed. Once the patient has sat down on the edge of the bed, ask them to put their right forearm onto the bed. If this is a profiling bed, raise the head of the bed a little, but not too far up as this will prevent the patient from getting into bed. If it is a non-profiling bed, put pillow(s) in place. Adopt a walk stance position while you do this (Figure 27.1).

2   Ask the patient to bring their left leg up onto the bed. Ask them to keep their head forward. Put your hand where you want their head to be and ask them to aim their forehead towards it. This will keep the patient's left shoulder forward and prevent them from falling back onto the bed (Figure 27.2).

3   Once the patient has their left leg on the bed, ask them to bring their right leg up. This needs to be carried out at the patient's pace and they should not be rushed (Figure 27.3).

4   Once both legs are on the bed the patient can start to swivel round (Figure 27.4).

5.   Continue with the manoeuvre in small movements until the patient is fully on the bed (Figures 27.5 a and b).

6   Once this manoeuvre has been completed, re-assess to ensure that they are capable of carrying out this task again with this level of intervention. If not, there may need to be two handlers or the introduction of equipment. Many patients have difficulty getting their legs into bed. See Chapter 41, Moving a patient's legs into bed with a slide sheet, for more information. If the patient cannot move themselves up the bed it may be necessary to use a slide sheet. See Chapter 36, Moving a semi-independent patient up the bed on a roller slide sheet.

After the task

1   Check that the patient has no pain and/or discomfort and is in the correct position on the bed.

2   Raise the bed rails if indicated in the handling plan and there has been an up-to-date bed rails assessment form completed.

3   Put the bed at a height that is safe for the patient.

28 Standing a patient up from the bed edge

Figure 28.1   Sit beside the patient with both of your feet flat on the floor and your arm across their back

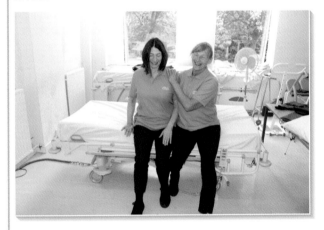

Figure 28.2   If you cannot reach across their back, place your hand in the middle of their back

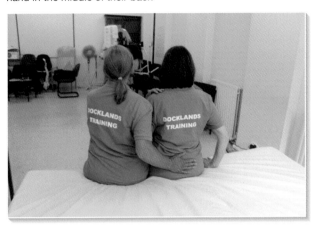

Figure 28.3   Place your outer hand on the patient's shoulder

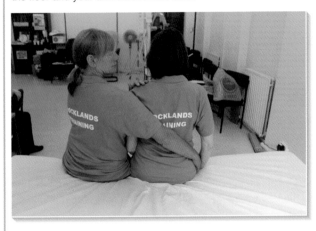

Figure 28.4   The patient's hands should be on the bed and their thigh

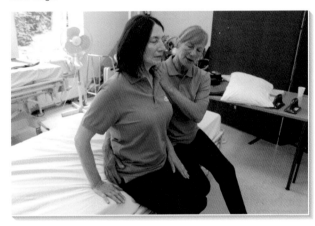

Figure 28.5   Using clear instructions, stand up from the bed together

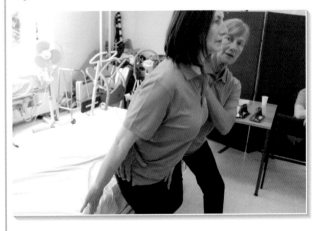

Figure 28.6   Stay close to the patient until they are stable

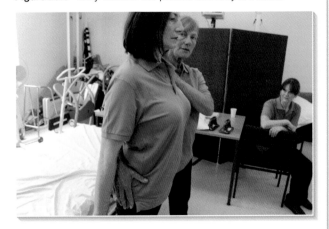

Purpose

To safely stand a patient up from a bed while maintaining a good posture.

Prior to the handling task

1 Consult any handling plans relating to this patient and check that they are clear, up-to-date and regularly reviewed.

2 If there is no written plan, ask your colleagues if they have relevant information relating to this patient.

3 Ensure a suitable and sufficient assessment has been carried out beforehand.

4 Communicate with the patient and tell them what you plan to do. Ensure that they understand and obtain their consent.

5 Make a final check that the patient cannot do this for themselves before continuing with the task.

6 Ensure that the patient is at the edge of the bed and has good sitting balance.

During the task

1 Sit beside the patient on the bed. Ensure that your feet are in a walk stance position with your feet facing in the direction you are going. Ask the patient to put one foot in front of the other. If the patient has a weakness on one side, check again if it is safe to stand them; if so, ensure their strong leg is placed back and the weak leg is placed forward. You will need to stand on the weak side. If necessary get the help of another handler to stand on the opposite side.

2 Place your hand nearest the patient onto the opposite iliac crest (Figure 28.1). If this involves too much stretching, put your hand in the centre of the lower back below the waist line (Figure 28.2).

3 Place your hand furthest away from the patient in front of the patient's shoulder. One of the patient's hands is placed on the bed and the other on their thigh (Figures 28.3 and 28.4).

4 Using clear verbal instructions such as 'Ready, Steady, Stand', or other verbal prompts agreed with the patient, ask the patient to stand up, bringing their head forward with their nose coming over their toes. One of the patient's hands pushes on the bed and the other pushes on their thigh. The patient should be leading the move with you guiding.

- Do not rock the patient unless it had been identified in the risk assessment that this is necessary (Figure 28.5).

5 If the patient is continuing to have difficulty, then stop and re-assess. It may be necessary to introduce a piece of handling equipment, for example a standing hoist. See Chapter 53, Use of a standing hoist.

6 When the patient is standing stay close by them, keeping your hand around their back and your hand on the shoulder until they are steady (Figure 28.6).

7 Offer them your hand that is on the shoulder in a palm to palm grip with thumbs tucked in. See Section 7 and Figure 16.6 of 'During the task' in Chapter 16, Standing a patient from a chair, for more information.

8 If appropriate hand the patient their walking frame. If you are using a walking frame ensure that it is in good condition and is the correct height for the patient. See Chapter 21, Tips for using walking frames and further information.

After the task

1 Check that the patient is safe and comfortable.

2 Document if the patient experiences any dizziness, light-headedness or other conditions that may put them at risk.

29 Standing a patient up from the bed edge using a profiling bed

Figure 29.1 The patient's feet must be flat on the floor as they sit on the edge of the bed

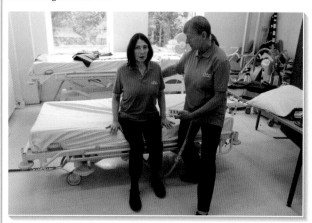

Figure 29.2 You will raise the bed using the correct button – the third one down in this picture

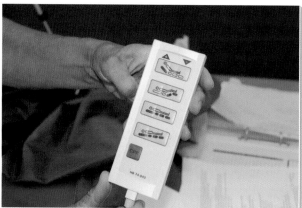

Figure 29.3 Ask the patient to move their head forward and push on the bed

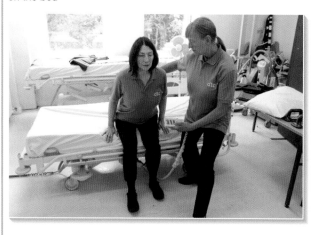

Figure 29.4 Gradually raise the bed. The patient must transfer their weight into their legs

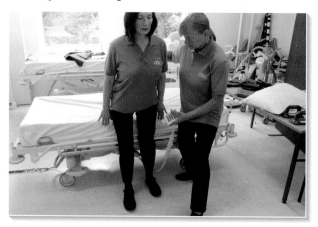

Figure 29.5 (a, b) Continue until the patient is standing

(a)

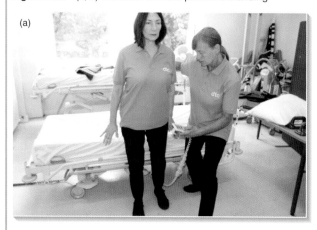

(b)

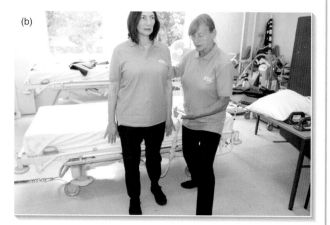

Moving and Handling Patients at a Glance. First Edition. Hamish MacGregor. © 2016 John Wiley & Sons, Ltd. Published 2016 by John Wiley & Sons, Ltd.

Purpose

To safely stand up a patient from a bed whilst maintaining a good posture.

Prior to the handling task

1   Consult any handling plans relating to this patient. Check that they are clear, up-to-date and regularly reviewed.
2   If there is no written plan ask your colleagues if they have relevant information relating to this patient.
3   Ensure a suitable and sufficient assessment has been carried out beforehand.
4   Communicate with the patient and tell them what you plan to do. Ensure that they understand and obtain their consent.
5   Make a final check that the patient cannot do this for themselves before continuing with the task.
6   Ensure that the patient is at the edge of the bed and has good sitting balance.

During the task

1   Ask the patient to sit at the edge of the bed with their feet flat on the floor in a step stance position. Ensure that you have a good posture and have a stable mobile base of support (Figure 29.1).
2   With one hand on the patient's back and your finger on the up button of the profiling bed (this is the third button from the top of the handset in Figure 29.2), ask the patient to bring their nose over their toes and push up with their hands, which should be pressing on the bed (Figure 29.3).
3   Encourage the patient to stand straight as you gradually raise the bed. The patient must transfer their weight forward through their legs (Figure 29.4).

• If at this point the patient is not managing this, stop, move close to the patient and sit them back down on the bed.
• Depending on your assessment of the patient, it may be necessary to have another handler at the other side of the patient and start the manoeuvre again.
• Alternatively you may want to stand the patient up with two people using the technique described in Chapter 28, Standing a patient up from the bed edge.

4   If the patient is continuing to have difficulty, then stop and re-assess. It may be necessary to introduce a piece of handling equipment, for example a standing hoist. See Chapter 53, Use of a standing hoist.
5   Continue this gradual process until your patient is in a safe and stable standing position (Figures 29.5 and 29.6).
6   Some patients can manage this move on their own if they have been given instructions on how to use the bed controls and have been assessed as safe to do so.
7   If appropriate hand the patient their walking frame. If you are using a walking frame ensure that it is in good condition and is the correct height for the patient. See Chapter 21, Tips for using walking frames, and further information.

After the task

1   Check that the patient is safe and comfortable.
2   Document if the patient experiences any dizziness, light-headedness or other conditions that may put them at risk.

30 Turning a patient in bed: verbal

Figure 30.1 Ask the patient to bend their knee, place their hand on their shoulder and face you

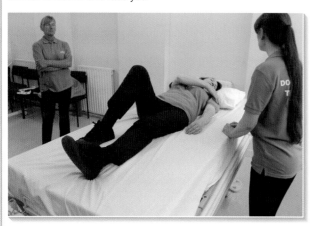

Figure 30.2 Encourage the patient to move onto their side

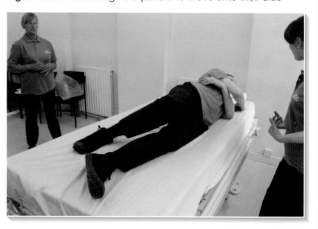

Figure 30.3 Use clear simple instructions to assist the patient

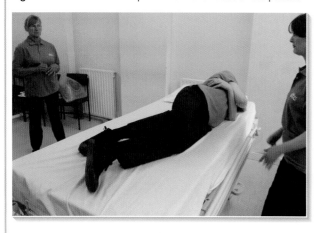

Figure 30.4 Alternatively you can ask the patient to bend both knees up

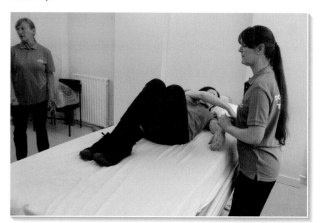

Figure 30.5 Bending both knees up may make it easier for the patient to turn onto their side

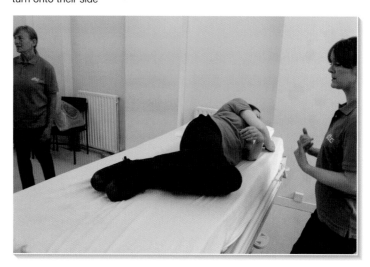

Moving and Handling Patients at a Glance. First Edition. Hamish MacGregor. © 2016 John Wiley & Sons, Ltd. Published 2016 by John Wiley & Sons, Ltd.

Purpose

To assist a patient to move onto their side by giving verbal prompts.

Prior to the handling task

1 Consult any handling plans relating to this patient and check that they are clear, up-to-date and regularly reviewed.

2 If there is no written plan, ask your colleagues if they have relevant information relating to this patient.

3 Communicate with the patient and tell them what you plan to do. Ensure that they understand and obtain their consent.

4 Ensure that the bed is at the correct height, that is, at waist height of the shorter handler.

During the task

1 Ask the patient to bend up their leg that is furthest away from you; their furthest away hand is then placed on their shoulder next to you, and their head is looking towards you (Figure 30.1).

2 Agree clear verbal prompts with the patient, such as 'Ready, Steady, Roll'. These are preferable to prompts such as 1, 2, 3 (see Chapter 6, Controversial techniques).

   • Having said this, if the patient is used to using 1, 2, 3, then it can be acceptable to use this as long as you and the patient are clear as to when the patient will turn.

   • The important thing is that you are encouraging the patient to move themselves.

   • Be aware that the patient may be anxious about moving and may require reassurance.

   • Do not place your hands on the patient, as the expectation is that the patient will do this activity themselves (Figures 30.2 and 30.3).

3 Alternatively, ask the patient to bend both knees up, as well as placing their hand nearest you on their opposite shoulder and their head looking towards you (Figure 30.4).

4 When the patient is ready, ask them to turn on the command that you have agreed with them.

5 If the patient has difficulty achieving the turn, ask them if they would like to try again. Give them sufficient time to prepare to try again.

6 Once the patient has moved onto their side, ensure that they are in a comfortable position (Figure 30.5).

7 If the patient is unable to turn in bed on their own, then they may have to be assisted by one person (see Chapter 31, Turning a patient in bed: one handler) or, assisted by two people (see Chapter 32, Turning a patient in bed: two handlers). It is important to assess the patient's need for assistance based on your moving and handling assessment rather than the patient not being given enough time to achieve this on their own.

8 Some things that may be preventing the patient from turning in bed in their own:

   • They do not understand what they need to do.
   • They are being rushed.
   • They are in pain.
   • They are on a pressure relieving mattress that is too soft.
   • They are anxious.
   • They are frightened.

These are only some examples; communicating clearly with the patient and assessing their needs may highlight other problems.

After the task

1 Check that the patient has no pain and/or discomfort.

2 Position them on their side with pillows or a positioning wedge for comfort.

3 Raise the bed rails if indicated in the handling plan, ensuring there has been an up-to-date bed rails assessment form completed.

4 Put the bed at a height that is safe for the patient.

31 Turning a patient in bed: one handler

Figure 31.1 Ensure the bed is at the correct height (i.e waist height of the handler)

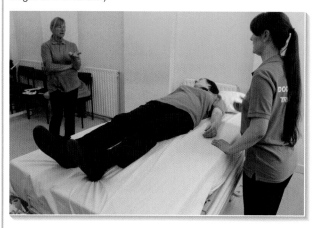

Figure 31.2 Ask patient to bend their knee, place their hand on their shoulder and face you

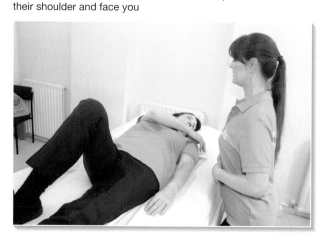

Figure 31.3 Place your hands on the patient's shoulder and hips without over-stretching

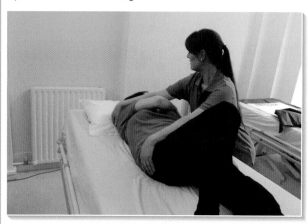

Figure 31.4 Adopting a walk stance position, turn the patient onto their side by transferring your weight from your front leg to your back leg

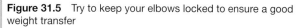

Figure 31.6 Once the patient has rolled, step back into the bed

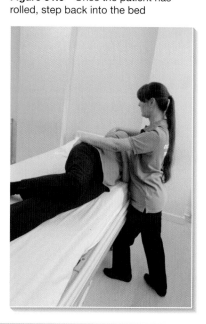

Figure 31.5 Try to keep your elbows locked to ensure a good weight transfer

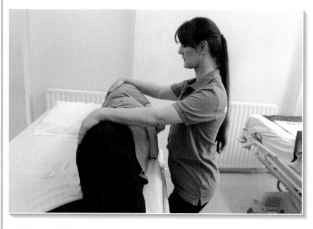

Moving and Handling Patients at a Glance. First Edition. Hamish MacGregor. © 2016 John Wiley & Sons, Ltd. Published 2016 by John Wiley & Sons, Ltd.

Purpose

To assist a patient to move onto their side.

Prior to the handling task

1 Consult any handling plans relating to this patient and check that they are clear, up-to-date and regularly reviewed.
2 If there is no written plan, ask your colleagues if they have relevant information relating to this patient.
3 Communicate with the patient and tell them what you plan to do. Ensure that they understand and obtain their consent.
4 Make a final check that the patient cannot do this for themselves before continuing with the task.
5 Ensure that the bed is at the correct height, that is, at waist height of the handler (Figure 31.1).

During the task

1 Ask the patient to bend up their leg that is furthest away from you; their furthest away hand is placed on their shoulder next to you and their head is looking towards you (Figure 31.2).
2 Adopt a walk stance position. Stand at the side of the bed so that your hands can easily be placed on the patient's shoulders and hips without over stretching (Figure 31.3).

  • If you are overstretching you will need to ask the patient to move closer to the edge of the bed nearest to you.
  • If the patient is unable to do this then you will need to enlist the help of a colleague to move the patient and/or use a piece of handling equipment such as a slide sheet.

3 Use clear verbal prompts such as 'Ready, Steady, Roll', or other verbal prompts agreed with the patient. See Chapter 30, Turning a patient in bed: verbal, for more information. Move the patient onto their side by transferring your weight from your front leg onto your back leg. At the same time keep your elbows locked (Figures 31.4 and 31.5).

  • If you find yourself bending your elbows, you are putting an excessive strain on your shoulder, neck and upper back.
  • This over time can lead to a cumulative musculoskeletal injury.

4 Once the patient has rolled on to their side, step closer to the bed so that you are next to the patient (Figure 31.6). This needs to be done speedily otherwise the patient may be fearful of the space between the edge of the bed and you.
5 Do not lean over side rails to turn a patient as this can cause over stretching and could contribute to cumulative musculoskeletal injury.

After the task

1 Check that the patient has no pain and/or discomfort.
2 Position them on their side with pillows or a positioning wedge for comfort.
3 Raise the bed rails if indicated in the handling plan, ensuring that there has been an up-to-date bed rails assessment form completed.
4 Put the bed at a height that is safe for the patient.

32 Turning a patient in bed: two handlers

Figure 32.1 Ensure that the bed is at your waist height

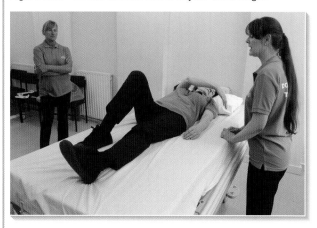

Figure 32.2 If the patient cannot bend either of their legs, place a pillow between them

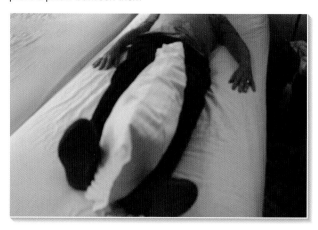

Figure 32.3 Adopting a walk stance position, place your hands on the patient's shoulders, hips and thighs

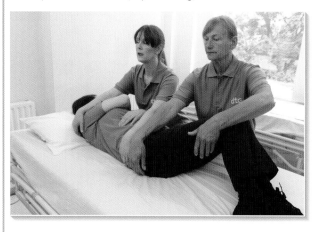

Figure 32.4 On the count of 'Ready, Steady, Roll', move the patient

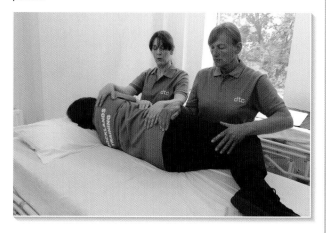

Figure 32.5 Transfer your weight from the front leg to the back leg

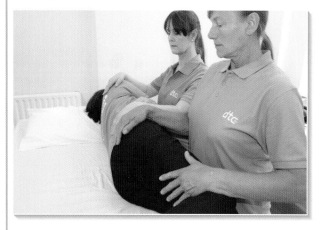

Figure 32.6 Once the patient has rolled, step back into the bed

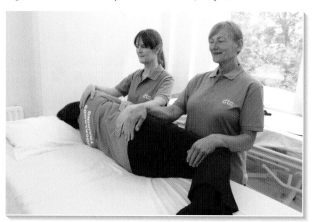

Moving and Handling Patients at a Glance. First Edition. Hamish MacGregor. © 2016 John Wiley & Sons, Ltd. Published 2016 by John Wiley & Sons, Ltd.

Purpose

To assist a patient to move onto their side with assistance.

Prior to the handling task

1   Consult any handling plans relating to this patient and check that they are clear, up-to-date and regularly reviewed.

2   If there is no written plan, ask your colleagues if they have relevant information relating to this patient.

3   Communicate with the patient and tell them what you plan to do. Ensure that they understand and obtain their consent.

4   Make a final check that the patient cannot do this for themselves before continuing with the task.

5   Ensure that the bed is at the correct height, that is, at waist height of the shorter handler.

During the task

1   Ask the patient to bend up their leg that is furthest away from you; their furthest away hand is placed on their shoulder next to you and their head is looking towards you (Figure 32.1).

2   If the patient cannot bend either of their legs, place a pillow between their legs as this will help the top leg to move over (Figure 32.2).

• Do not ask the patient to put one ankle on top of the other as this potentially puts strain on the patient's hip.

• If you are overstretching you will need to ask the patient to move closer to the edge of the bed nearer to you.

• If the patient is unable to do this then you will need to enlist help to move the patient and/or use a piece of handling equipment such as a slide sheet.

3   Adopt a walk stance position. Position yourselves at the side of the bed so that your hands can be easily placed on the patient's shoulders, hips and thighs without overstretching (Figure 32.3).

4   Use clear verbal prompts such as 'Ready, Steady, Roll', or other verbal prompts agreed with the patient. See Chapter 30, Turning a patient in bed: verbal, for more information. Move the patient onto their side by transferring your weight from your front leg onto your back leg. At the same time keep your elbows locked (Figure 32.4).

• If you find yourself bending your elbows you are putting an excessive strain on your shoulder, neck and upper back.

• This over time can lead to musculoskeletal injury.

5   Once the patient has rolled onto their side, step closer to the bed so that you are next to the patient (Figures 32.5 and 32.6).

• This needs to be done speedily otherwise the patient may be fearful of the space between the edge of the bed and you.

6   Do not lean over side rails to turn a patient as this can cause over stretching of the lower back and could contribute to cumulative musculoskeletal injury.

After the task

1   Check that the patient has no pain and/or discomfort.

2   Position them on their side with pillows or a positioning wedge for comfort.

3   Raise bed rails if indicated in the handling plan ensuring there has been an up-to-date bed rails assessment form completed.

4   Put the bed at a height that is safe for the patient.

33 Inserting two flat slide sheets under a patient: unravelling technique

Figure 33.1 Fold both slide sheets together with the handles on each sheet facing outwards

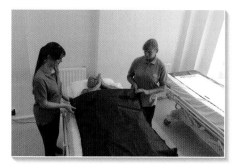

Figure 33.2 The folds should be about a hand width apart. Then place under the pillow with the open ends on top (see Figure 33.4)

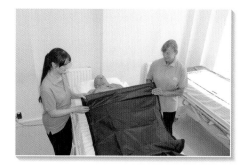

Figure 33.3 Both handlers should face the head of the bed with inside palm up and thumb tucked in

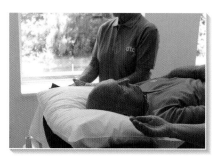

Figure 33.4 The inner hand goes under and grips the bottom section and the outer hand the top

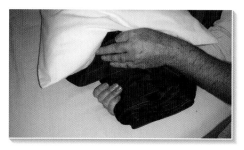

Figure 33.5 Adopt a walk stance position; keeping elbows on the bed, pull the bottom section down

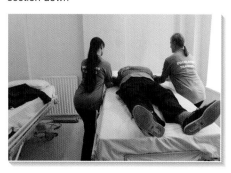

Figure 33.6 Both handlers should ensure that they work in unison as the slide sheet is unravelled

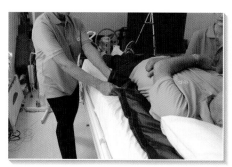

Figure 33.7 As the slide sheet goes under the patient, the outer hand can be removed

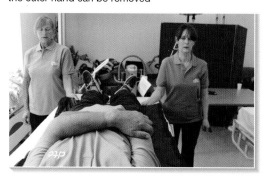

Moving and Handling Patients at a Glance. First Edition. Hamish MacGregor. © 2016 John Wiley & Sons, Ltd. Published 2016 by John Wiley & Sons, Ltd.

Purpose

To move a patient up the bed who is unable to do so.

Prior to the handling task

1   Consult any handling plans relating to this patient and check that they are clear, up-to-date and regularly reviewed.

2   If there is no written plan, ask your colleagues if they have relevant information relating to this patient.

3   Communicate with the patient and tell them what you plan to do. Ensure that they understand and obtain their consent.

4   Make a final check that the patient cannot do this for themselves before continuing with the task.

5   Ensure that the bed is at the correct height, that is, at waist height of the shorter handler.

During the task

1   With the handlers at either side of the bed, fold the slide sheet over the patient with the handles of each slide sheet being up on the top sheet and down on the bottom sheet.

   • The folds should be about one hand width apart (Figures 33.1 and 33.2).

   • If you are unable to fold the slide sheet on top of the patient find another suitable surface to carry out this task.

   • If you are in hospital this is not on another bed as this will contravene infection control protocols.

2   Place the folded slide sheets under the patient's pillow with the open ends on top facing the head of the bed. This should be gently manoeuvred under the patient's shoulders.

3   Both handlers should face the head of the bed and have their inside hand palm up and thumb tucked in (Figure 33.3).

4   Adopt a walk stance position, and place their inside hand with thumb tucked in under the pillow and slide sheets. The handler's outer hand should take hold of the top part of the folded slide sheets (Figure 33.4).

5   The bottom sections of the slide sheets should be pulled down underneath the patient. The handlers must keep their elbows on the bed as this will prevent them from pulling the slide sheet up instead of down towards the bottom of the bed (Figures 33.5 and 33.6).

6   The handlers must communicate with each other as they unravel the slide sheets. Using verbal prompts such as 'Ready, Steady, Pull', will ensure that both handlers are working together. This needs to be continued until the slide sheet is fully under the patient. Once the slide sheet is under the patient's back, the handlers can remove their outer hand and adopt a better posture. The slide sheet will remain in position as it is anchored by the patient (Figure 33.7).

7   If the slide sheet gets stuck under the lumbar curve of the patient's back you can:

   a.   pull the slide sheet down on one side while the second handler keeps hold of their side. Repeat on the other side. This 'see-saw' action can help the slide sheet to go under the patient's hips;

   b.   push down on the mattress at the hips as the slide sheet is pulled under the patient;

   c.   bring the slide sheet from the feet rather than the shoulders. Be careful here as the slide sheet can get caught in the patient's clothing if this method is adopted.

After the task

1   Check that the patient has no pain and/or discomfort.

2   Prepare to move the patient in bed as necessary.

34 Inserting two flat slide sheets under the patient: by rolling patient

Figure 34.1   Put the slide sheets together, handles facing outwards

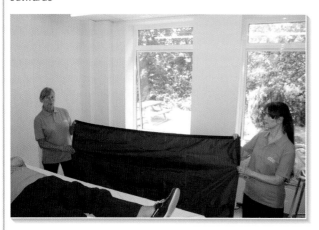

Figure 34.2   Fold one-third of the slide sheets over

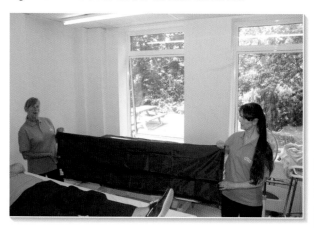

Figure 34.3   Fold into sections and place under the pillow

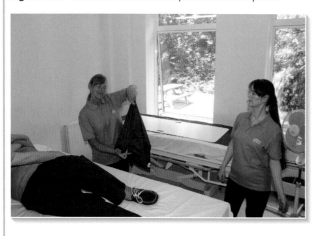

Figure 34.4   Unfold slide sheets and place at patient's back, with one-third underneath

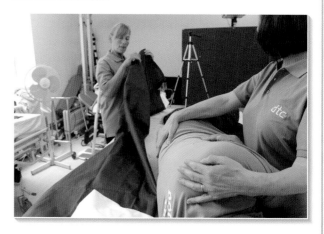

Figure 34.5   Allow patient to lie on their back, and pull the third section from under the neck

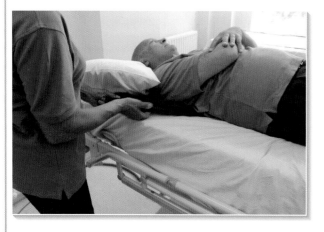

Figure 34.6   Gradually pull from the top and bottom until the slide sheets are fully through

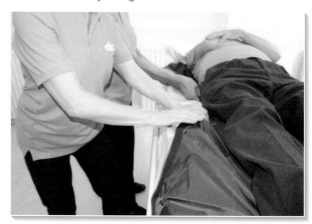

Moving and Handling Patients at a Glance. First Edition. Hamish MacGregor. © 2016 John Wiley & Sons, Ltd. Published 2016 by John Wiley & Sons, Ltd.

Purpose

To move a patient up the bed who is unable to do so.

Prior to the handling task

1   Consult any handling plans relating to this patient and check that they are clear, up-to-date and regularly reviewed.

2   If there is no written plan, ask your colleagues if they have relevant information relating to this patient.

3   Communicate with the patient and tell them what you plan to do. Ensure that they understand and obtain their consent.

4   The patient needs to turn on their side. An assessment needs to be made as to whether the patient can do this for themselves or with the assistance of one or two handlers. See Chapter 30, Turning a patient in bed: verbal; Chapter 31, Turning a patient in bed: one handler; or Chapter 32, Turning a patient in bed: two handlers, for alternatives.

Ensure that the bed is at the correct height, that is, at waist height of the shorter handler.

During the task

1   The two slide sheets are placed together with the handles facing outwards (Figure 34.1).

2   One-third of the slide sheets are folded as shown in Figure 34.2.

3   The pair of slide sheets are then folded into sections so that they can be placed next to the patient without them coming apart (Figure 34.3).

• This allows both handlers to have their hands free to help the patient if necessary.

• Placing the folded slide sheets under the patient's pillow is one of the easiest places to store them temporarily.

4   Turn the patient on their side as described in Chapters 30, 31 or 32, based on the dependency level of the patient.

5   The slide sheets are then placed behind the patient's back, the one-third fold underneath with that fold next to the patient's back (Figure 34.4).

6   The handler at the opposite side of the bed can place their hands under the patient to pull the remaining slide sheet through under the patient.

• It is often easiest to start at the foot of the bed by pulling the slide sheet under the patient's legs, then when you reach the hips move to the head of the bed.

• Start to pull the slide sheet from under the patient's neck and work your way down the patient's body (Figure 34.5).

7   This is repeated until the whole slide sheet is under the patient. The second handler may assist in this process (Figure 34.6).

• Please note that these are small gentle pulls and you need to adopt a walk stance position and use your body weight to pull out the slide sheet.

• Avoid using bent elbows as this puts strain on the shoulders, neck and upper back and over time can lead to cumulative musculoskeletal injury.

After the task

1   Check that the patient has no pain and/or discomfort.

2   Prepare to move the patient up the bed as described in Chapter 38, Moving a patient up the bed with two flat slide sheets; or on their side as described in Chapter 40, Turning a patient in bed with flat slide sheets.

35 Inserting a roller slide sheet under a patient

Figure 35.1 Folded slide sheet with open ends at the side for moving the patient up the bed

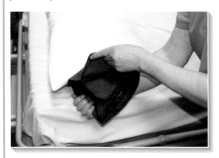

Figure 35.2 Folded slide sheet with open ends at the top for moving the patient on their side

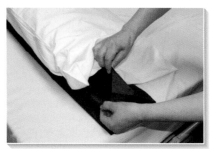

Figure 35.3 Place folded slide sheets under the patient's pillow

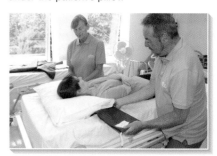

Figure 35.4 Your outer hand should grip the top part of the folded sheet; your inner hand the bottom

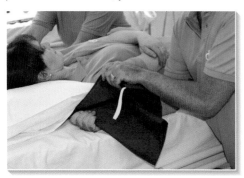

Figure 35.5 Pull the bottom section of the slide sheet under the patient. Do this in unison with your partner

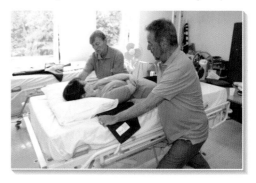

Figure 35.6 Keep your elbow on the bed as you do this

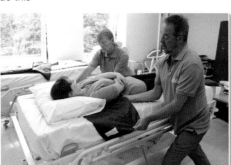

Figure 35.7 Once the slide sheet is under the patient's back, you can remove your outer hand

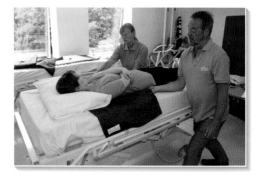

Figure 35.8 Continue down the bed

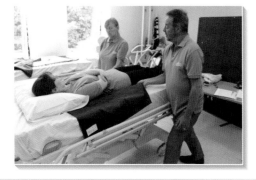

Figure 35.9 Be aware of your posture as you continue to pull through the slide sheet

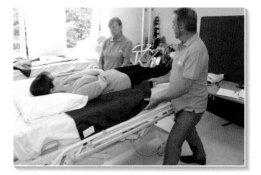

Moving and Handling Patients at a Glance. First Edition. Hamish MacGregor. © 2016 John Wiley & Sons, Ltd. Published 2016 by John Wiley & Sons, Ltd.

Purpose

To move a patient up the bed who is unable to assist.

Prior to the handling task

1 Consult any handling plans relating to this patient and check that they are clear, up-to-date and regularly reviewed.

2 If there is no written plan, ask your colleagues if they have relevant information relating to this patient.

3 Communicate with the patient and tell them what you plan to do. Ensure that they understand and obtain their consent.

4 Make a final check that the patient cannot do this for themselves before continuing with the task.

5 Ensure that the bed is at the correct height, that is, at waist height of the smaller handler.

During the task

Unravelling technique

1 With the handlers at either side of the bed, fold the slide sheet with the open ends at the side if the patient is to be moved up the bed (Figure 35.1).

- If the patient is to be turned on their side in bed the open ends of the slide sheet must be at the top (Figure 35.2).
- The folds should be about one hand width apart.
- See Chapter 33, Inserting two flat slide sheets under a patient: unravelling technique, for pictures of how to fold up the sheet.

2 Place the folded slide sheets under the patient's pillow. This should be gently manoeuvred under the patient's shoulders (Figure 35.3).

3 Both handlers should face the head of the bed, adopt a walk stance position, and place their inside hand with thumb tucked in under the pillow and slide sheet. The handler's outer hand should take hold of the top part of the slide sheet (Figure 35.4).

4 The bottom section of the slide sheet should be pulled down underneath the patient. The handler must keep their elbow on the bed as this will prevent them from pulling the slide sheet up as well instead of down towards the bottom of the bed (Figure 35.5).

5 This needs to be continued until the slide sheet is fully under the patient. Once the slide sheet is under the patient's back the handler can remove their outer hand and adopt a better posture. The slide sheet will remain in position as it is anchored by the patient (Figures 35.6, 35.7, 35.8 and 35.9).

Insertion by rolling the patient

1 Turn the patient on their side as described in Chapter 30, Turning a patient in bed: verbal; Chapter 31, Turning a patient in bed: one handler; or Chapter 32, Turning a patient in bed: two handlers, based on the dependency level of the patient.

2 Roll the slide sheet in half and place at the patient's back. If possible place as much of the slide sheet as possible under the patient's legs.

- The way the slide sheet is inserted will depend on the direction that the patient needs to be moved. (see Figures 35.1 and 35.2).

3 Roll the patient onto their back, and if possible pull the remaining slide sheet through under the patient.

4 If the patient is large, then it will be necessary to roll the patient in the opposite direction as above and then pull the slide sheet through.

After the task

1 Check that the patient has no pain and/or discomfort.

2 Prepare to move the patient in bed as necessary.

36 Moving a semi-independent patient up the bed with a roller slide sheet

Figure 36.1 Encourage the patient to move to allow the slide sheet to be put under the patient's shoulders and hips

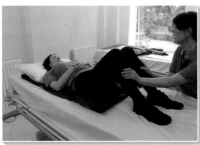

Figure 36.2 Ask the patient to bend their knees

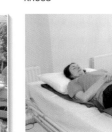

Figure 36.3 Ask the patient to push their feet

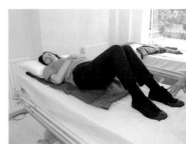

Figure 36.4 If necessary, place your hands on the lower limbs

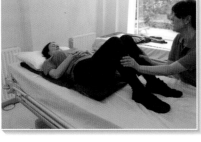

Figure 36.5 Do not put your hands on the patient's ankles

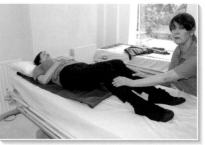

Figure 36.6 If the patient is unable to help, put your hand between the slide sheet and pull through

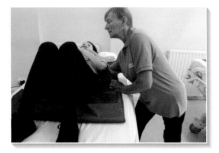

Figure 36.7 Pull a small section of the slide sheet through

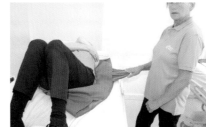

Figure 36.8 Continue to pull through using both hands

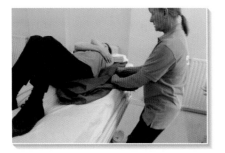

Figure 36.9 Continue until completely removed

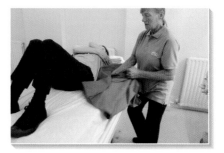

Moving and Handling Patients at a Glance. First Edition. Hamish MacGregor. © 2016 John Wiley & Sons, Ltd. Published 2016 by John Wiley & Sons, Ltd.

Purpose

To move a patient up the bed who needs minimal assistance.

Prior to the handling task

1 Consult any handling plans relating to this patient and check that they are clear, up-to-date and regularly reviewed.

2 If there is no written plan, ask your colleagues if they have relevant information relating to this patient.

3 Communicate with the patient and tell them what you plan to do. Ensure that they understand and obtain their consent.

4 Make a final check that the patient has the ability to carry out this technique. The patient will need:

- to have the ability to follow simple instructions;
- to have strength in their legs;
- to have their pain well controlled and minimised.

5 Ensure that the bed is at the correct height, that is, at waist height of the shorter handler.

6 If the bed is an electric profiling bed then the head section will need to be put flat.

During the task

1 Insert the slide sheet by either method described in Chapter 35, Inserting a roller slide sheet under a patient. Alternatively the patient may be able to roll themselves from side to side to allow the slide sheet to be inserted. The slide sheet needs to have the open ends at either side of the bed. As this patient only needs minimal assistance they are likely to be able to move side to side to allow you to insert the slide sheet (Figure 36.1).

2 Encourage the patient to bend their knees and with their feet flat on the bed push themselves up the bed (Figures 36.2 and 36.3).

3 If the patient finds this difficult, then place your hands on the patient's lower limbs (Figure 36.4) and encourage them to move themselves up the bed (Figure 36.5). DO NOT put your hands on the patient's ankles as this will impede their ability to move up the bed. This is because the patient needs to be able to push their heels into the bed to carry out this manoeuvre.

4 If the patient is unable to turn from side to side to allow you to remove the slide sheet, then the slide sheet can be removed by the handler putting their hand under the patient's lower back and taking hold of the bottom part of the slide sheet on the opposite side of the bed (Figure 36.6).

5 The slide sheet is pulled through under the patient with the handler adopting a walk stance position and using a weight transfer movement; the slide sheet is removed with slow steady pulls (Figure 36.7).

6 It is important to get a small piece of the slide sheet that you can use with both hands and using a 'see-saw' movement the slide sheet will come out without causing any tissue viability problems to the patient (Figures 36.8 and 36.9).

After the task

1 Check that the patient has no pain and/or discomfort.

2 Raise the bed rails if indicated in the handling plan ensuring there has been an up-to-date bed rails assessment form completed.

3 Put the bed at a height that is safe for the patient.

37 Moving a patient up the bed with a roller slide sheet

Figure 37.1   Place a small slide under the patient's heels

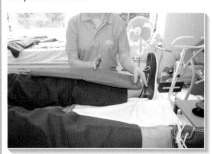

Figure 37.2   If the patient cannot help, 'scissor' slide sheet under each ankle

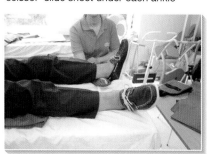

Figure 37.3   Adopting a walk stance position, hold the top part of the slide sheet with your inner hand

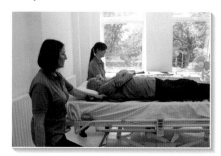

Figure 37.4   In a coordinated way, move the patient a small distance up the bed using a weight transfer

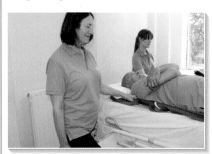

Figure 37.5   Remove the small slide sheet

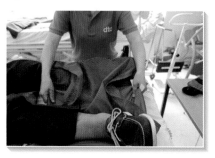

Figure 37.6   Remove by pulling the slide sheet from underneath

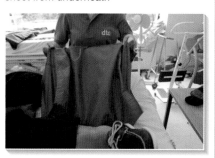

Figure 37.7   Place your hand under the patient's knees and grip the bottom part of the slide sheet

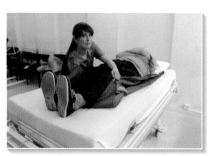

Figure 37.8   Pull through gradually using both hands

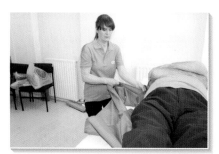

Moving and Handling Patients at a Glance. First Edition. Hamish MacGregor. © 2016 John Wiley & Sons, Ltd. Published 2016 by John Wiley & Sons, Ltd.

Purpose

To move a patient up the bed who is unable to do so.

Prior to the handling task

1   Consult any handling plans relating to this patient and check that they are clear, up-to-date and regularly reviewed.
2   If there is no written plan, ask your colleagues if they have relevant information relating to this patient.
3   Communicate with the patient and tell them what you plan to do. Ensure that they understand and obtain their consent.
4   Make a final check that the patient cannot do this for themselves before continuing with the task.
5   Ensure that the bed is at the correct height, that is, at waist height of the shorter handler.

During the task

1   Insert the slide sheet by one of the methods described in Chapter 35, Inserting a roller slide sheet under the patient. The most appropriate method will be determined by your assessment of the patient.
2   The slide sheet needs to have the open ends at either side of the bed.
3   A small roller slide sheet should be placed under the patient's heels as this will reduce friction when the patient is moved up the bed and reduce the risk of tissue damage. This can be done by 'scissoring' the folded slide sheet under the patient's nearest ankle then pulling the slide sheet through and repeating the process under the second ankle (Figures 37.1 and 37.2).

4   The handlers should then stand at the top of the bed facing the bottom of the bed. Adopting a walk stance, take a position with the hand closest to the bed, taking hold of the top part of the slide sheet in an overhand grip (Figure 37.3).
5   On the command of 'Ready, Steady, Move', both handlers weight transfer and slowly move the patient up the bed no more than 2 cm (1 inch) (Figure 37.4). The handlers continue to do this until the patient has reached the desired position in the bed.
6   Once the patient is in the desired position the small roller slide sheet is removed from under the heels by pulling it under itself. This will ensure that there is no friction on the patient's skin (Figures 37.5 and 37.6).
7   Then the roller slide sheet is removed from under the patient by one of the handlers placing their inside hand under the patient's knees and taking hold of the bottom part of the slide sheet on the opposite side of the bed (Figure 37.7). The slide sheet is pulled through under the patient with the handler adopting a walk stance position, and using a weight transfer movement the slide sheet is removed with slow steady pulls (Figure 37.8).
8   It is important to grasp a small piece of the slide sheet that you can use with both hands and using a 'see-saw' movement the slide sheet will come out without causing any tissue viability problems to the patient.

After the task

1   Check that the patient has no pain and/or discomfort.
2   Raise the bed rails if indicated in the handling plan ensuring there has been an up-to-date bed rails assessment form completed.
3   Put the bed at a height that is safe for the patient.

38 Moving a patient up the bed with two flat slide sheets

Figure 38.1 Adopting a walk stance position, hold the top slide sheet with your inner hand

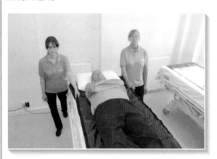

Figure 38.2 In a coordinated way, move the patient a small distance up the bed using a weight transfer

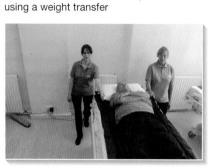

Figure 38.3 Continue until the patient is in the desired position

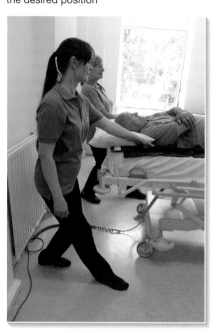

Figure 38.4 If the head of the bed can be removed, stand at the head of the bed

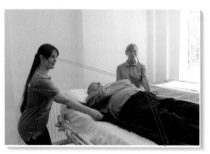

Figure 38.5 If using both hands, grip the top slide sheet at the patient's shoulders and hips

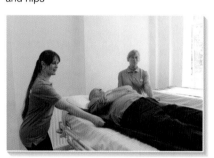

Figure 38.6 If using both hands, you must look at the opposite corner of the bed

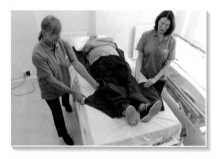

Figure 38.7 Remove the slide sheets by pulling under from opposite corners

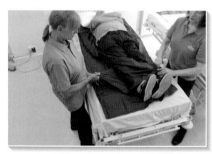

Figure 38.8 Keep your hands close to the patient as the slide sheet is removed

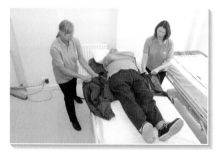

Figure 38.9 Remove the slide sheets in unison

Moving and Handling Patients at a Glance. First Edition. Hamish MacGregor. © 2016 John Wiley & Sons, Ltd. Published 2016 by John Wiley & Sons, Ltd.

Purpose

To move a patient up the bed who is unable to do so.

Prior to the handling task

1   Consult any handling plans relating to this patient and check that they are clear, up-to-date and regularly reviewed.
2   If there is no written plan, ask your colleagues if they have relevant information relating to this patient.
3   Communicate with the patient and tell them what you plan to do. Ensure that they understand and obtain their consent.
4   Make a final check that the patient cannot do this for themselves before continuing with the task.
5   Ensure that the bed is at the correct height, that is, at waist height of the shorter handler.

During the task

1   Insert the slide sheet using either method described in Chapter 33, Inserting two flat slide sheets under the patient: unravelling technique; or Chapter 34, Inserting two flat slide sheets under the patient: by rolling the patient.
2   The handlers should then stand at the head of the bed facing the bottom of the bed. Adopting a walk stance position with the hand closest to the bed taking hold of the top part of the slide sheet in an overhand grip (Figure 38.1).
3   On the command of 'Ready, Steady, Move', both handlers weight transfer and slowly move the patient up the bed no more than 2 cm (1 inch) (Figure 38.2).
4   The handlers continue to do this until the patient has reached the desired position in the bed (Figure 38.3).

5   **Alternative method 1:** If the head of the bed can be removed, the handlers can stand at the head of the bed and adopting a walk stance position move the patient up the bed using the technique described previously (Figure 38.4).
6   **Alternative method 2:** The handlers can use both hands in an overhand grip at the patient's hip and shoulders, then move the patient up the bed as described previously (Figure 38.5). If this method is employed the handlers must look at the bottom of the bed diagonally opposite (Figure 38.6).
7   Remove the slide sheets by each handler going to the foot of the bed and taking the opposite corner of the slide sheet and pulling it underneath. This will ensure that the slide sheet slides on itself and does not damage the patient's skin (Figure 38.7).
8   Each handler adopts a walk stance position and using their body weight pulls the slide sheet towards them. This must be done in unison and using verbal prompts such as 'Ready, Steady, Pull', will ensure that this happens. The handlers must keep their hands close to the patient to ensure that the slide sheets slide under each other (Figure 38.8).
9   The handlers walk up the bed and steadily pull out the slide sheet. This is done with slow steady pulls, not by short sharp pulls. This is continued until both slide sheets are removed from under the patient (Figure 38.9).

After the task

1   Check that the patient has no pain and/or discomfort and is in the correct position in the bed.
2   Raise the bed rails if indicated in the handling plan ensuring there has been an up-to-date bed rails assessment form completed.
3   Put the bed at a height that is safe for the patient.

39 Turning a patient in bed with roller slide sheets

Figure 39.1 Lower the bed to hip height

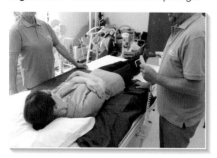

Figure 39.2 Adopt a walk stance position with hips and knees bent and grip the top of the slide sheet

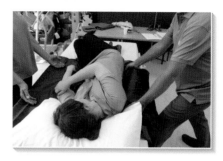

Figure 39.3 Grip the top slide sheet at the patient's hips and shoulders and pull it towards you

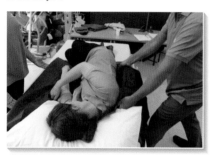

Figure 39.4 Keep moving your hands closer to the patient as you pull the slide sheet until the patient is on their side

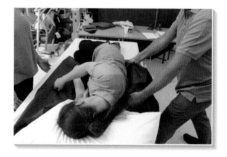

Figure 39.5 Remove the slide sheet by gripping the bottom part of the slide sheet next to the patient's back

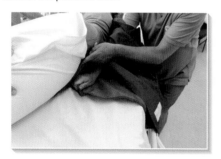

Figure 39.6 In a walk stance position, transfer your body weight back

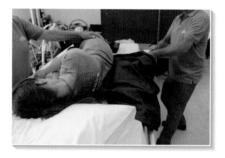

Figure 39.7 Remove the slide sheet by pulling it through gradually

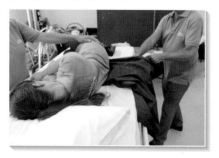

Figure 39.8 The slide sheet should be 'outside in' when it is fully removed

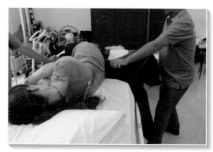

Moving and Handling Patients at a Glance. First Edition. Hamish MacGregor. © 2016 John Wiley & Sons, Ltd. Published 2016 by John Wiley & Sons, Ltd.

Purpose

To turn a patient in bed who is unable to do so, while keeping them in the centre of the bed.

Prior to the handling task

1   Consult any handling plans relating to this patient and check that they are clear, up-to-date and regularly reviewed.
2   If there is no written plan, ask your colleagues if they have relevant information relating to this patient.
3   Communicate with the patient and tell them what you plan to do. Ensure that they understand and obtain their consent.
4   Make a final check that the patient cannot do this for themselves before continuing with the task.
5   Ensure that the bed is at the correct height, that is, at waist height of the shorter handler.

During the task

1   Insert the slide sheet by one of the methods described in Chapter 35, Inserting a roller slide sheet under the patient. The slide sheet needs to have the open ends facing the top and bottom of the bed and is under the patient's shoulders and hips.
2   The handlers should be at either side of the bed. (A third handler may need to be available to assist in turning the patient.)
3   Ask the patient to bend their leg that is closest to you up; their nearest hand is placed on the shoulder away from you and their head looking way from you. If necessary the handlers may have to assist the patient to do this.

4   Lower the bed to thigh height (Figure 39.1). This will allow the handler to use their leg muscles rather than their arm muscles to carry out the manoeuvre. The handler adopts a walk stance position with their hips and knees bent, and takes hold of the top slide sheet in an overhand grip (Figure 39.2).
5   Keeping hands next to the patient the handler moves the top slide sheet upwards no more than 2 cm. The handler must move from hips and knees and keep their elbows locked (Figure 39.3).
6   As the patient moves, the handler moves their hands closer to the patient (Figure 39.4) and repeats the movement.
7   This is repeated until the patient is on their side. *This is a series of small gentle, slow moves.*
8   Once the patient is in the optimum position, the slide sheets are removed. The bed must be brought up to the waist height of the handler removing the slide sheet. The handler removes the slide sheet from behind the patient's back, taking hold of the bottom part of the slide sheet (Figure 39.5). The slide sheet is pulled through under the patient with the handler adopting a walk stance position, and using a weight transfer movement the slide sheet is removed with slow steady pulls (Figures 39.6, 39.7 and 39.8).

After the task

1   Check that the patient has no pain and/or discomfort.
2   Insert a pillow or a positioning wedge if necessary to keep the patient in position.
3   Raise the bed rails if indicated in the handling plan and there has been an up-to-date bed rails assessment form completed.
4   Put the bed at a height that is safe for the patient.

40 Turning a patient in bed with two flat slide sheets

Figure 40.1 Lower the bed to hip height and grip the slide sheet at patient's hips and shoulders

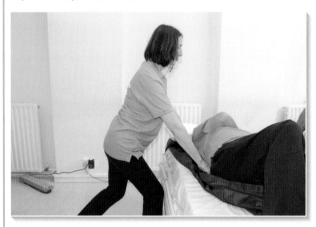

Figure 40.2 Adopt a walk stance position with hips and knees bent and pull the slide sheet towards you

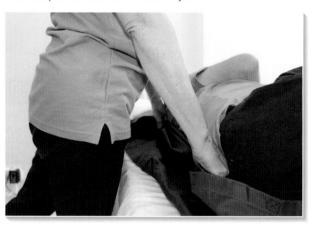

Figure 40.3 Keep moving your hands closer to the patient as you pull the slide sheet

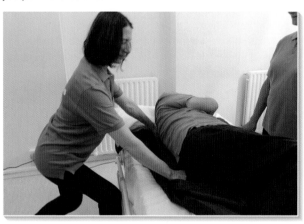

Figure 40.4 Once the patient is in the desired position move the bed up to waist height

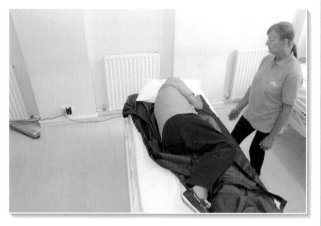

Figure 40.5 The slide sheets are removed one at a time by pulling the top slide sheet under itself

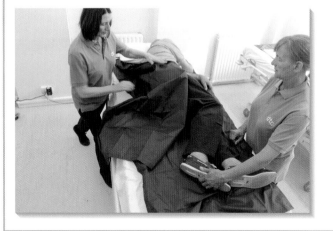

Figure 40.6 The bottom slide sheet is removed in a similar way

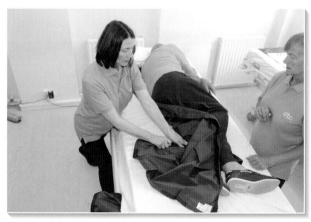

Moving and Handling Patients at a Glance. First Edition. Hamish MacGregor. © 2016 John Wiley & Sons, Ltd. Published 2016 by John Wiley & Sons, Ltd.

Purpose

To turn a patient in bed who is unable to do so, while keeping them in the centre of the bed.

Prior to the handling task

1 Consult any handling plans relating to this patient, checking that they are clear, up-to-date and regularly reviewed.

2 If there is no written plan, ask your colleagues if they have relevant information relating to this patient.

3 Communicate with the patient and tell them what you plan to do. Ensure that they understand and obtain their consent.

4 Make a final check that the patient cannot do this for themselves before continuing with the task.

5 Ensure that the bed is at the correct height, that is, at waist height of the shorter handler.

During the task

1 Insert the slide sheets as described in Chapter 33, Inserting two flat slide sheets under the patient: unravelling method; or Chapter 34, Inserting two flat slide sheets under the patient: by rolling the patient.

2 The handlers should be at either side of the bed. (There may be need for a third handler to be available to assist in turning the patient.)

3 Ask the patient to bend their leg up that is closest to you; their nearest hand is placed on the shoulder away from you and their head looking away from you. If necessary the handlers may have to assist the patient to do this.

4 Lower the bed to thigh height. This will allow the handler to use their leg muscles rather than their arm muscles to carry out the manoeuvre. The handler adopts a walk stance position with their hips and knees bent (Figure 40.1).

5 Grip the top slide sheet in an overhand grip (Figure 40.2).

6 Keeping your hands next to the patient the handler moves the top slide sheet upwards no more than 2 cm. The handler must move from hips and knees and keep their elbows locked (Figure 40.3).

7 As the patient moves onto their side, the handler moves their hands closer to the patient and repeats the movement.

8 This is repeated until the patient is on their side. This is a series of small gentle, slow moves.

9 Once the patient is in the optimum position, the slide sheets are removed. The bed must be brought up to the waist height of the handler before doing this (Figure 40.4).

10 The slide sheets must be removed one at a time from the patient's back as this will prevent the patient from rolling onto their back again. One handler moves to the foot of the bed. The top slide sheet is folded under itself and removed by the handler adopting a walk stance position and using a weight transfer movement removing the slide sheet by a series of slow steady pulls (Figure 40.5).

11 This is repeated to remove the bottom slide sheet (Figure 40.6).

After the task

1 Check that the patient has no pain and/or discomfort.

2 Insert a pillow or a positioning wedge if necessary to keep the patient in position.

3 Raise the bed rails if indicated in the handling plan ensuring there has been an up-to-date bed rails assessment form completed.

4 Put the bed at a height that is safe for the patient.

41 Moving a patient's legs into bed with a slide sheet

Figure 41.1 Fold the slide sheet with the handles up on the long section and down on the bottom section

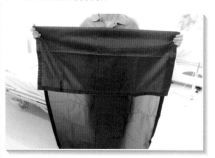

Figure 41.2 Place the slide sheet on the bed with the edge of the bottom section a hand width from the edge of the bed

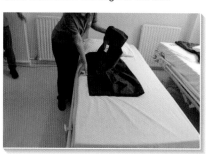

Figure 41.3 Tuck the long section under the mattress slightly

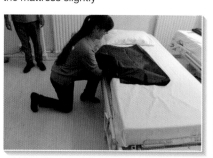

Figure 41.4 Ask the patient to sit on the bed and remove the long section from under the mattress

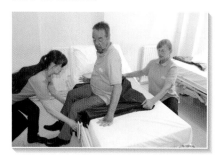

Figure 41.5 Take the slide sheet by the handles at the patient's ankles

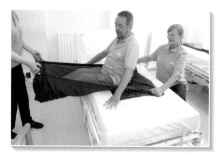

Figure 41.6 Keep the patient's legs close to you as you move them onto the bed

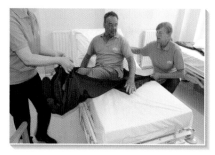

Figure 41.7 The patient can slide themselves up the bed

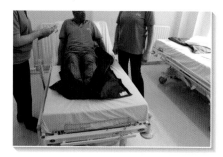

Figure 41.8 Remove the slide sheet by folding it under itself

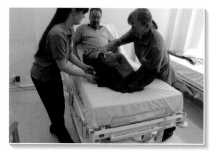

Figure 41.9 Pull under using slow gentle movements

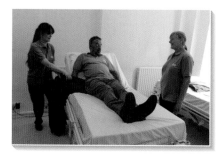

Moving and Handling Patients at a Glance. First Edition. Hamish MacGregor. © 2016 John Wiley & Sons, Ltd. Published 2016 by John Wiley & Sons, Ltd.

Purpose

To move a patient's legs into bed with a flat slide sheet with handles. This technique *will not work* with a flat slide sheet *without handles*.

Prior to the handling task

1 Consult any handling plans relating to this patient checking that they are clear, up-to-date and regularly reviewed.

2 If there is no written plan, ask your colleagues if they have relevant information relating to this patient.

3 Communicate with the patient and tell them what you plan to do. Ensure that they understand and obtain their consent.

4 Make a final check that the patient cannot do this for themselves before continuing with the task.

5 The patient must be mobile enough to have walked to the bed. They must have good cognition and have upper body strength and trunk control. They must be able to use their arms.

6 This technique is *not suitable for someone with very heavy legs*.

During the task

1 Fold the slide sheet over with the handles facing up on the long section of slide sheet and facing down on the short section (Figure 41.1).

2 Put the slide sheet on the bed as shown in Figure 41.2. There must be a section at the side of the bed where the slide sheet is not doubled over. *This is essential as there is the potential for them to slide off the bed when they sit down.*

3 Tuck the long section loosely under the mattress so that it does not create a slipping hazard for the patient (Figure 41.3).

4 Ask the patient to sit down and position themselves in the centre of the slide sheet with the back of their knees on the edge of the mattress. If this is an electric profiling bed then the back-rest should be raised. The patient must support themselves with their arms; their hands should be placed on the mattress NOT the slide sheet. The handler begins to take the long section of the slide sheet from beneath the mattress (Figure 41.4).

5 The handler then pulls out the long section of slide sheet so that it cocoons the patient's legs. Grasping the handles where the patient's ankles are located in the slide sheet, move the patient's legs towards the bed. The legs must be kept close to the handler and they must ensure they maintain a good posture as they carry out this technique. A second handler should be behind the patient to ensure that they do not fall backwards (Figures 41.5 and 41.6).

6 Once the patient is in the bed they can move themselves up the bed by pushing their hands into the bed. The handlers should ensure that the bed is at the correct height for themselves as they may have to carry out additional handling. See point 8 below (Figure 41.7).

7 The slide sheet can be removed by the patient lifting their hips off the bed.

8 Alternatively the slide sheet can be folded underneath itself from the bottom of the bed, and using slow gentle movements the handler pulls the slide sheet out as they move towards the top of the bed (Figures 41.8 and 41.9).

After the task

1 Check that the patient has no pain and/or discomfort.

2 Raise the bed rails if indicated in the handling plan ensuring there has been an up-to-date bed rails assessment form completed.

3 Put the bed at a height that is safe for the patient.

42 Types of hoist

Figure 42.1 Types of mobile hoists

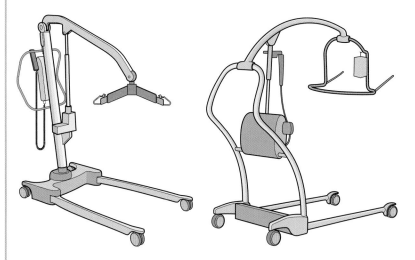

Figure 42.2 Ceiling track hoist

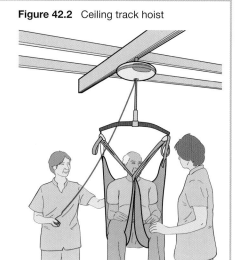

Figure 42.3 Gantry hoist

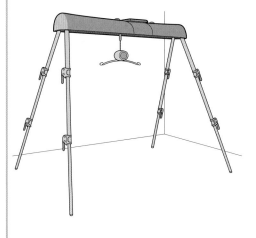

Figure 42.4 Types of standing hoists

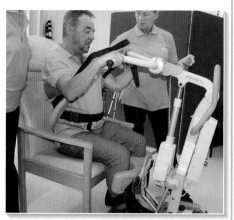

Figure 42.5 (a) Bed head, (b) bath, and (c) pool hoist

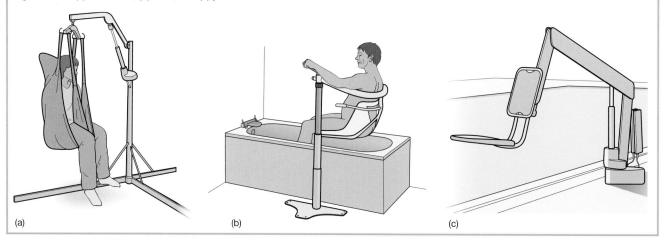

(a)   (b)   (c)

Moving and Handling Patients at a Glance. First Edition. Hamish MacGregor. © 2016 John Wiley & Sons, Ltd. Published 2016 by John Wiley & Sons, Ltd.

There are many different type of hoist on the market and it is important that before you use a hoist you ensure that you are familiar with the controls and functions.

The vast majority of hoists are electrical which means that they are either plugged into the mains to charge or there is a separate battery that is charged in a separate charging unit. There are still a small number of hydraulic hoists that are powered by hand using a lever that is pumped.

You should have been shown how to use the hoist before you attempt to use it; ideally you should have read the instruction leaflet that comes with the hoist. There are often abridged instructions that come with a hoist; these can be laminated and attached to the hoist.

Your checklist should include:
- Is the hoist in a good general condition?
- Is the hoist clean?
- Is the hoist charged?
- Does the spreader bar move smoothly up and down?
- Where is the emergency stop?
- Where is the emergency lower?
- Will the hoist take the weight of the patient?
- Has the hoist been inspected by a competent person in the past 6 months?
- If it is a mobile hoist do the wheels move smoothly and do the feet open out?
- If it is a ceiling tracking hoist or a gantry hoist does the hoist unit move smoothly along the track? In addition a ceiling tracking hoist may have to be returned to a charging point along the rail; failure to do this might mean the hoist will be unavailable to be used for the next patient transfer.

Type of hoist

Mobile hoists (Figure 42.1)

These come in various sizes and shapes and are the most common type of hoist seen both in the hospital and in the community. These hoists have various weight capacities ranging from 120 kg up to 320 kg. See Chapter 59, Use of equipment for bariatric patients. These can be used anywhere because they are portable but can be difficult to move when:
- The patient is heavy.
- The flooring is uneven or carpeted.
- There is a confined space.

For more information on the use of these hoists, see Chapters 51–53.

Ceiling tracking hoists (Figure 42.2)

These are installed into the ceiling with a tracking system. This can be a simple track or a movable H frame that allows the tracking to cover a whole room. There are also systems that can move the patient from one room into another such as from bedroom to bathroom. Some systems allow tracking to be installed and the hoisting unit to be attached as needed. This is useful in nursing homes where the hoisting needs of the residents may vary.

The advantage of this type of hoist is that it does not require a large piece of machinery to be moved around as the hoisting unit is just brought down from the ceiling. The disadvantage is that the hoist will only operate as far as the tracking will reach.

Gantry hoists (Figure 42.3)

These are similar to the ceiling tracking hoist, but are suspended from a frame erected over the area that the hoisting procedure is carried out. This means that there is no structural intervention to install the track which can be costly. The system is portable and can be dismantled when no longer needed, but does mean that the area available for hoisting can be quite limited usually from bed to chair. The community setting is where these hoists are more commonly used.

Standing hoists (Figure 42.4)

These are used when the patient must have some weight bearing ability, trunk control and the ability to cooperate and follow instructions. They are often used as part of a patient's rehabilitation. See Chapter 53, Using a standing hoist, for more information.

Bed head hoists (Figure 42.5a)

These are simple hoists that are attached at the head of the bed and are used in people's homes where space is at a premium. The hoist is fixed so is limited to move as far as the swing of the arm of the hoist. The maximum use would be to hoist a patient from bed to chair.

Bath hoists (Figure 42.5b)

These are used to hoist a patient in and out of the bath and often used in conjunction with a variable height bath.

Pool hoists (Figure 42.5c)

These are used either in swimming pools or hydrotherapy pools to hoist a person in and out of the water.

43 Types of sling

Figure 43.1 Loop type sling

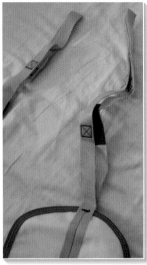

Figure 43.2 Clip type sling

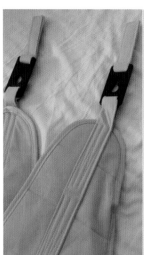

Figure 43.3(a) Clip type spreader bar

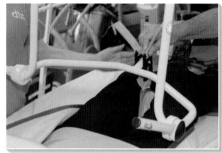

(b) Loop type spreader bar

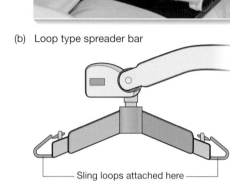

Sling loops attached here

Figure 43.4 Quick fit sling

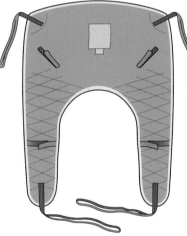

Figure 43.5 Quick fit deluxe sling

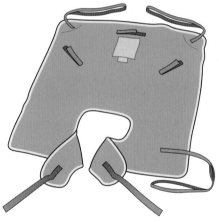

Figure 43.6 Toileting/access sling

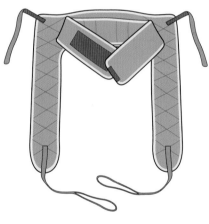

Figure 43.7 *In situ* or all day sling

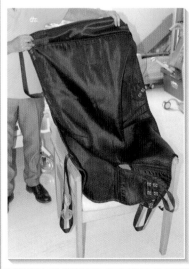

Figure 43.8 Stretcher sling

Moving and Handling Patients at a Glance. First Edition. Hamish MacGregor. © 2016 John Wiley & Sons, Ltd. Published 2016 by John Wiley & Sons, Ltd.

There are a huge number of slings available and this is just an overview of the types of slings that are available.

If you are in anyway unsure about the sling that you are using then stop and seek advice. Before using any sling you need to carry out some checks. These are fully explained in the next chapter (Chapter 44, Insertion of sling into bed – 'Prior to the handling task' section).

Sling sizes

Slings come in all sizes from some for small children through to bariatric patients. As well as checking the maximum weight of the patient for the sling, the sling needs to be the correct size for the patient. A sling that is too large will allow the patient's hips to slide through the aperture and a sling that is too small will be painful as it crushes the patient. Measuring the correct size of sling is a skilled task and should not be undertaken without having achieved the correct level of competence. This can only be achieved with face to face training. Most sling manufacturers provide guidance on how to measure for their particular sling.

Sling types

Disposable slings and slings that can be laundered

Disposable slings are thrown away after the patient no longer needs the sling, it is soiled or it is damaged. The patient's name should be marked on the sling to prevent it from being shared with other patients.

Slings that can be laundered must be kept clean and must not be shared with other patients. In addition to being checked before use they are subject to the Lifting Operations and Lifting Equipment Regulations (1998) which states that they are examined by a competent person at 6-monthly intervals. This check should be marked on a label attached to the sling.

Loop slings and clip slings

These describe the way that the sling is attached to the spreader bar of the hoist.

Figure 43.1 is a loop type sling and Figure 43.2 is a clip type sling.

Figure 43.3 illustrates both types of spreader bar.

Loops go with loops and clips go with clips. **The two cannot be mixed.**

Head supports

Slings can come with or without head supports and the patient's risk assessment should identify if a head support is necessary.

General purpose universal sling often called a 'Quick Fit Sling'

This comes in both loops and clips. This type of sling offers the patient a good level of support. There is an example of this in Figure 43.4. The loop needs to be attached in a way that allows the patient to be hoisted in the optimum functional position that is comfortable and maintains dignity. For example, if the patient needs to be in a seated position the shoulder straps of the sling should be on a short loop and the leg straps should be on a longer loop, 'short shoulders – long legs' because of its simple design, this sling is relatively easy to fit.

Quick Fit Deluxe Sling

This is a loop sling that has additional leg loops that give the patient increased comfort and support (Figure 43.5). This type of sling by its nature is more difficult to fit as there are extra loops to attach

Toileting or access sling

This type of sling has less material and therefore is quite easy to fit (Figure 43.6). The leg straps are attached as above but the shoulder straps are lower down and are under the patient's arms with a strap that is attached around the patient's waist. The patient *must* have upper body strength and sitting balance and good cognition to use this sling. The sizing must be accurate, as a sling that is too large will allow the patient to slide through the sling and be held under the arms causing damage similar to that of a drag lift (see Chapter 6, Controversial techniques).

In situ or all day slings

These slings are designed to be left under the patient as it not acceptable to leave a standard sling under a patient. These are made in material that allows the air to flow though and there are a minimum of seams. They often have pockets for the loops to go into so that they do not cause skin damage. An example of this is shown in Figure 43.7.

Stretcher slings

These allow the patient to be flat lifted from the bed (Figure 43.8). This can be useful for patients with fractures or complex health care needs.

44 Insertion of sling into bed

Figure 44.1 Fold the sling in half with the labels and handles on the outside

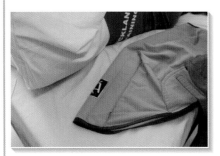

Figure 44.2 Place the sling along the patient's back leaving a 5 cm/2 inch gap (approx)

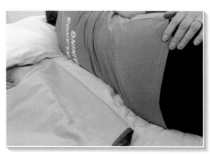

Figure 44.3 Take the leg piece and place under the pillow beneath the patient's neck

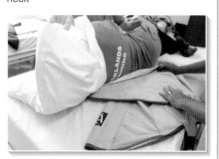

Figure 44.4 Fold the top part of the sling in a big roll into the patient's back

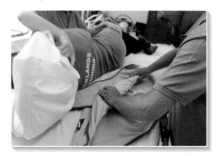

Figure 44.5 Allow the patient onto their back and pull the leg piece from under the pillow toward the foot of the bed

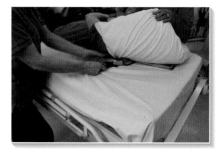

Figure 44.6 Using a weight transfer technique pull the leg piece fully down

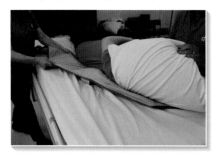

Figure 44.7 Ask the patient to lift their leg and place the leg piece underneath

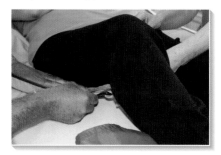

Figure 44.8 If the patient cannot lift their leg, push the leg piece into the mattress with the loop or clip underneath

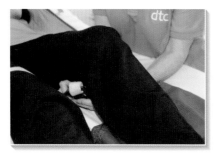

Figure 44.9 Alternatively move the patient's leg up using a small slide sheet under the ankles

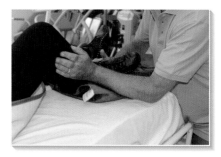

Purpose

To insert a sling under patient while in bed.

Prior to the handling task

1   Consult any handling plans relating to this patient and check that they are clear, up-to-date and regularly reviewed.
2   If there is no written plan, ask your colleagues if they have relevant information relating to this patient.
3   Communicate with the patient and tell them what you plan to do. Ensure that they understand and obtain their consent.
4   Check that the sling is in good order. Check for rips, loose stitching, cleanliness and general condition.
5   Check that the sling has a safe working load that can take the patient.
6   If it is a disposable sling, ensure that it is the patient's allocated sling and that their name is on it. Check that it has not previously got wet and that the safety label is intact.
7   If it is a reusable sling, check that it has been LOLER (Lifting Operation and Lifting Equipment Regulations, 1998) checked. See Chapter 2, Legislation II. It should have been checked every six months.
8   Ensure that the bed is at the correct height, that is, at waist height of the smaller handler.

During the task

1   Roll the patient on to their side in accordance with their abilities. See Chapter 30, Turning a patient in bed: verbal; Chapter 31, Turning a patient in bed: one handler; or Chapter 32, Turning a patient in bed: two handlers, for alternatives.
2   The handler folds the sling in half with the labels and straps to the outside (Figure 44.1).
3   Place the sling behind the patient about 2 cm from their back (Figure 44.2). The shoulder straps of the sling should be in line with the patient's shoulders.

4   Take the top leg piece and fold it up under the patient's neck beneath the pillow (Figure 44.3).
5   Roll the remainder of the sling over itself in big rolls until it is by the patient's back. Fill in the 2 cm space (Figure 44.4).
6   Allow the patient to roll onto their back.
7   The second handler pulls the leg piece from beneath the pillow and firmly pulls it down towards the foot of the bed (Figure 44.5).
8   The handler should adopt a walk stance position and transfer their weight as they carry out this task.
 • This will ensure that they use their hips and thigh muscles and their body weight, not their arms (Figure 44.6).
9   The position of the sling should then be checked.
 • It must be central under the patient.
 • Do not pull the sling into place as this can cause damage to the patient skin.
 • If the sling needs repositioning take it out as shown in Chapter 45, Removal of sling from bed, and re-insert.
10   The leg pieces are then inserted under the patient's legs. If the patient can raise one or both of their legs then the leg piece is placed under the leg (Figure 44.7).
11   If the patient is unable to lift their leg then the leg piece is bent underneath itself with the loop or clip underneath and it is pushed into the mattress and under the patient's leg (Figure 44.8).
12   Alternatively you can place a small slide sheet under the patient's heel and using a weight transfer move the patient's leg up to create a space to remove the sling (Figure 44.9).

After the task

1   Check that the patient has no pain and/or discomfort.
2   Check the sling in the correct position.

45 Removal of sling from bed

Figure 45.1 Ask the patient if they can bend their leg to allow you to remove the leg pieces

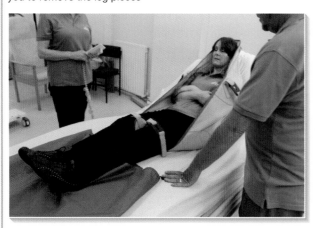

Figure 45.2 You can place a small slide sheet under the patient's heels to assist them to move their leg

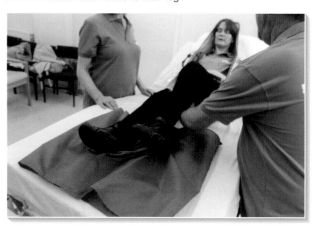

Figure 45.3 With the patient on their side, fold the leg piece underneath the sling

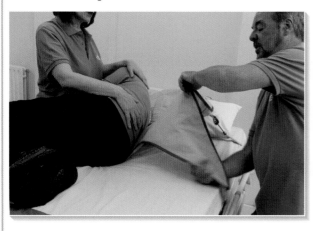

Figure 45.4 The leg piece should go under the patient's neck

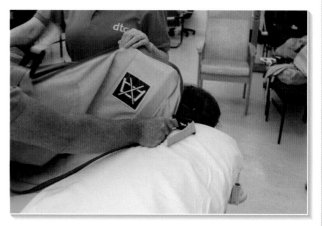

Figure 45.5 Roll the remaining sling under itself into the patient's back

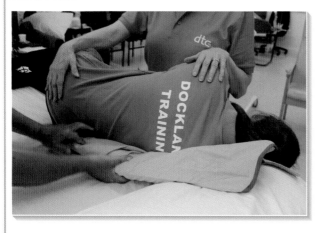

Figure 45.6 Once the patient is on their back, the leg piece is pulled through and out

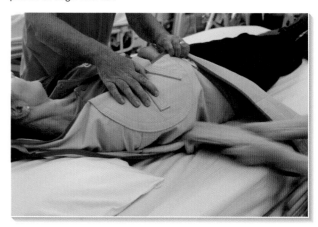

Moving and Handling Patients at a Glance. First Edition. Hamish MacGregor. © 2016 John Wiley & Sons, Ltd. Published 2016 by John Wiley & Sons, Ltd.

Purpose

To remove a sling from under the patient while in bed.

Prior to the handling task

1   Consult any handling plans relating to this patient, and check that they are clear, up-to-date and regularly reviewed.

2   If there is no written plan, ask your colleagues if they have relevant information relating to this patient.

3   Communicate with the patient and tell them what you plan to do. Ensure that they understand and obtain their consent.

4   Ensure that the bed is at the correct height, that is, at waist height of the smaller handler.

During the task

1   With a handler at each side of the bed, inform the patient that you are going to remove the leg pieces of the sling from under their thighs.

• Ask the patient to bend their knee upwards thus creating a space for the handler to remove the leg piece of the sling.

• If there is a problem with this, place a small slide sheet under the patient's heel and using a weight transfer move the patient's leg up to create a space to remove the sling (Figures 45.1 and 45.2).

2   When removing the leg piece ensure you roll it under itself to reduce the risk of tissue viability problems.

3   Roll the patient on their side in accordance with their abilities. See Chapter 30, Turning a patient in bed: verbal; Chapter 31, Turning a patient in bed: one handler; or Chapter 32, Turning a patient in bed: two handlers, for alternatives.

4   Fold the leg piece of the sling under the main part of the sling and place it under the patient's neck and pillow (Figures 45.3 and 45.4).

5   Roll the remainder of the sling under itself in big rolls until it is nested to the patient's back (Figure 45.5).

6   Allow the patient to roll onto their back. Warn the patient that there will be a large roll of sling under their back for a few seconds until the sling is removed.

7   The second handler pulls the leg piece from beneath the pillow and firmly pulls it down towards the foot of the bed.

• The handler should adopt a walk stance position and transfer their weight as they carry out this task.

• Slow gentle pulling of the sling is necessary to remove it.

• Do not tug sharply on the sling as this will be uncomfortable for the patient but also put excessive strain on the handler's back (Figure 45.6).

After the task

1   Check that the patient has no pain and/or discomfort.

2   Raise bed rails if indicated in the handling plan ensuring there has been an up-to-date bed rails assessment form completed.

3   Put the bed at a height that is safe for the patient.

46 Insertion of sling into chair

Figure 46.1 Ask the patient to sit forward and place a sling at the base of their back

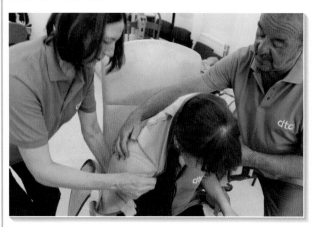

Figure 46.2 Bring the leg pieces around the patient. Keep your hand between the sling and the patient

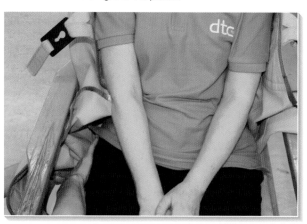

Figure 46.3 Once the sling is in place, ask the patient to lift their leg to insert the leg piece

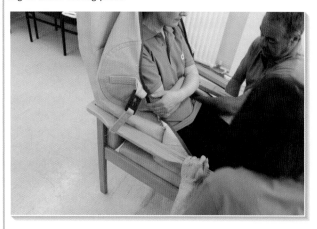

Figure 46.4 If the patient cannot lift their leg, ask them to lean to one side

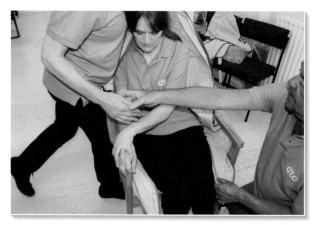

Figure 46.5 When the patient has moved to one side, the leg piece can be put under the patient's leg

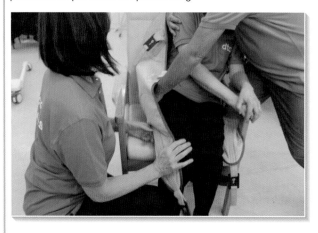

Figure 46.6 Keep your hand between the sling and the patient to minimise shearing

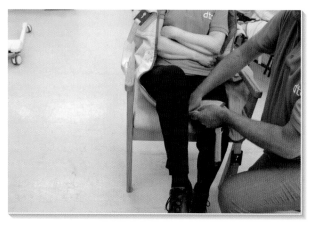

Moving and Handling Patients at a Glance. First Edition. Hamish MacGregor. © 2016 John Wiley & Sons, Ltd. Published 2016 by John Wiley & Sons, Ltd.

Purpose

To insert a sling under the patient while in a chair.

Prior to the handling task

1   Consult any handling plans relating to this patient and check that they are clear, up-to-date and regularly reviewed.

2   If there is no written plan, ask your colleagues if they have relevant information relating to this patient.

3   Communicate with the patient and tell them what you plan to do. Ensure that they understand and obtain their consent.

4   Check that the sling is in good order. Check for rips, loose stitching, cleanliness and general condition.

5   Check that the sling has a safe working load that can take the patient.

6   If it is a disposable sling, ensure that it is the patient's allocated sling and that their name is on it. Check that it has not previously got wet and that the safety label is intact.

7   If it is a reusable sling check that it has been LOLER (Lifting Operation and Lifting Equipment Regulations (1998)) checked. See Chapter 2, Legislation II. It should have been checked every six months.

During the task

1   Ask the patient to sit forward in the chair, if they are able. Then place the sling down the patient's back so that it reaches the bottom of their back. It does not need to go under their buttocks (Figure 46.1).

- If the patient is having difficulty in sitting forward then you can assist them by placing your hand behind the patient's shoulder and assisting them to sit forward.
- If you are still having difficulty, make use of a small roller slide sheet as described in Chapter 49, Insertion of a sling into chair with slide sheets.

2   Bring the leg pieces round the side of the patient's thighs. Place your hand between the sling and the patient to ensure the patient's skin is not harmed (Figure 46.2).

3   Continue one side at a time until the leg pieces are equal at both sides of the patient's thighs (Figure 46.3).

- Ask the patient to lift their legs one at a time to get the leg pieces under each leg.
- If they are unable to do this you can ask them to lean to one side of the chair to allow you to place the leg piece under the thigh (Figure 46.4).

4   Alternatively you can assist the patient to lean to one side while the other handler inserts the sling under the patient's thigh (Figure 46.5).

5   When inserting the sling under the patient's thigh, keep your hand between the sling and the patient's thigh and ensure any straps or clips are kept away from the patient's skin (Figure 46.6).

6   Check that the sling has no wrinkles or folds, as that can harm the patient, before attaching the hoist to the sling.

After the task

1.   Check that the patient has no pain and/or discomfort.

2.   Check the sling in the correct position.

47 Removal of sling from chair

Figure 47.1 Ask the patient to lift their leg and remove the leg piece by pulling it underneath

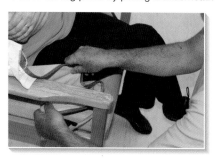

Figure 47.2 Move each leg piece along the side of the chair

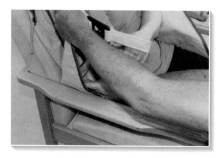

Figure 47.3 Fold the leg piece behind the sling at the patient's back

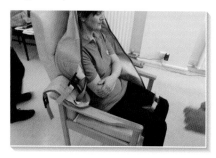

Figure 47.4 If the patient has difficulty in lifting their leg, insert a small slide directly under their leg

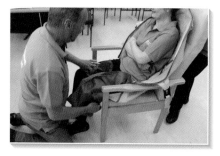

Figure 47.5 Place your hand under the patient's leg and hold the loop or clip of the sling

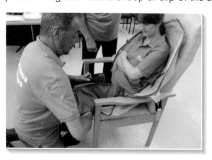

Figure 47.6 Pull the leg piece from underneath away from the patient

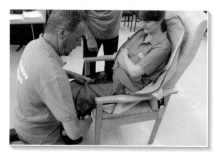

Figure 47.7 Encourage the patient to sit forward and pull the leg pieces upwards

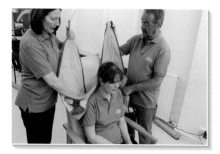

Figure 47.8 Working in unison, remove the sling

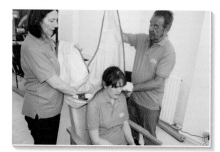

Moving and Handling Patients at a Glance. First Edition. Hamish MacGregor. © 2016 John Wiley & Sons, Ltd. Published 2016 by John Wiley & Sons, Ltd.

Purpose

To remove a sling from under the patient while they are in the chair. This is important, because unless the sling is designed to be left underneath the patient, then it must be removed. See Chapter 43, Types of sling – see 'in situ or all day' sling section for exceptions to this rule.

Prior to the handling task

1   Consult any handling plans relating to this patient and check that they are clear, up-to-date and regularly reviewed.
2   If there is no written plan, ask your colleagues if they have relevant information relating to this patient.
3   Communicate with the patient and tell them what you plan to do. Ensure that they understand and obtain their consent.
4   Ensure that you are in a good posture at the side of the patient's chair.

During the task

1   Ask the patient to lift their leg and fold the leg piece of the sling under itself away from the patient's skin. This is important to prevent skin damage (Figure 47.1).
2   Take the leg piece of the sling (always coming underneath) and move it along the side of the chair towards the back of the chair (Figure 47.2).

3   You should now have the leg piece folded behind the back of the sling at the back of the chair next to the patient's lower back (Figure 47.3).
4   Repeat the above on the patient's other leg.

If the patient is unable to lift their leg:

1   Slide a small roller slide sheet under the patient's leg (Figure 47.4).
2   Put your hand under the patient's knee and take hold of the loop or the clip of the sling (Figure 47.5).
3   Pull this underneath the patient's leg (folding underneath as shown previously) (Figure 47.6).
4   Continue to move the leg piece towards the back of the chair as shown previously.
5   Remove the slide sheet and repeat on the other side if necessary.
6   When both leg pieces are at the back of the chair encourage the patient to sit as far forward as they can. Pull the leg pieces behind the back of the sling, that is, the leg pieces are between the chair and the back of the sling NOT the patient. This needs the handlers working in unison so that both leg pieces come out at the same time (Figure 48.7).
7   Continue to do this until the sling in removed completely (Figure 47.8).

After the task

Check that the patient has no pain and/or discomfort.

48 Insertion of sling into bed with slide sheets

Figure 48.1 Take the sling with the handles and labels downwards

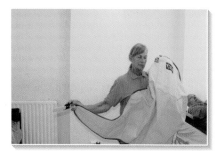

Figure 48.2 One handler pushes the leg piece under the arch in the patient's back between the slide sheets

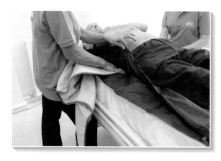

Figure 48.3 The second handler pulls the leg piece through and down slightly

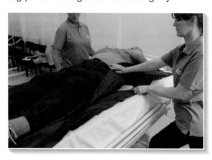

Figure 48.4 The first handler takes the shoulder strap and pushes between the slide sheets under the patient's neck

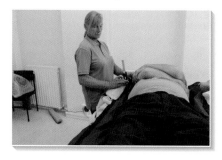

Figure 48.5 The second handler pulls the shoulder strap through

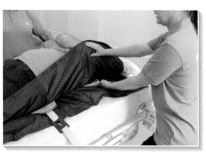

Figure 48.6 While the first handler holds the top slide sheet, the second handler pulls the sling through fully

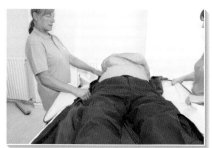

Figure 48.7 The top slide sheet can be removed by folding it under itself

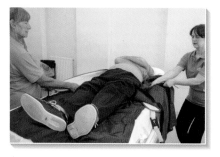

Moving and Handling Patients at a Glance. First Edition. Hamish MacGregor. © 2016 John Wiley & Sons, Ltd. Published 2016 by John Wiley & Sons, Ltd.

Purpose

To insert a hoist sling under a patient in bed who is unable to roll on to their side.

Before the technique

1　Consult any handling plans relating to this patient and check that they are clear, up-to-date and regularly reviewed.

2　If there is no written plan, ask your colleagues if they have relevant information relating to this patient.

3　Communicate with the patient and tell them what you plan to do. Ensure that they understand and obtain their consent.

4　Check that the sling is in good order. Check for rips, loose stitching, cleanliness and general condition.

5　Check that the sling has a safe working load that can take the patient.

6　If it is a disposable sling ensure that it is the patient's allocated sling and that their name is on it. Check that it has not previously got wet and that the safety label is intact.

7　If it is a reusable sling check that it has been LOLER (Lifting Operation and Lifting Equipment Regulations (1998)) checked. See Chapter 2, Legislation II. It should have been checked every six months.

8　Ensure that the bed is at the correct height, that is, at waist height of the smaller handler.

During the technique

1　Insert two flat slide sheets as described in Chapter 33, Inserting two flat slide sheets under a patient: unravelling technique.

2　There must be two handlers, one at either side of the bed.

3　Position the sling with all the labels and handles facing downward, that is, towards the floor (Figure 48.1).

4　Handler one takes the leg piece of the sling and places it under the small of the patient's back between the two slide sheets (Figure 48.2).

5　Handler two, who is on the opposite side of the bed, then takes the leg piece of the sling and pulls it through and slightly down. Do not pull too much of the sling through (Figure 48.3).

6　Handler one then takes the shoulder straps and puts it under the patient's neck between the two slide sheets (Figure 48.4).

7　Handler two takes the shoulder strap and pulls it through just enough to be visible from between the slide sheets (Figure 48.5).

8　Handler one takes hold of the top slide sheet as handler two gradually pulls the sling through until it is in the correct position. This should be carried out in slow controlled moves with the handler using their body weight to bring the sling through (Figure 48.6).

9　The sling can be gently adjusted by both handlers to ensure it is positioned correctly and that there are no creases.

10　The top slide sheet can be removed by folding it under itself and removed by the handler adopting a walk stance position and using a weight transfer to complete the removal (Figure 48.7).

11　The leg pieces can be slid under the patient's legs as in Chapter 44, Insertion of sling into bed (sections 10, 11 and 12).

12　When the sling is attached to the hoist, the bottom slide sheet is left behind on the bed.

After the task

1　Check that the patient has no pain and/or discomfort.

2　Check the sling is in the correct position.

49 Insertion of sling into chair with slide sheets

Figure 49.1 Place a small roller slide sheet behind the patient's shoulder

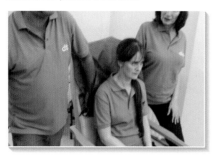

Figure 49.2 With your hands inside the slide sheet, in unison push down to the base of the patient's back

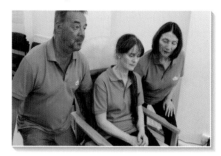

Figure 49.3 Take the sling and place between the slide sheet and the chair

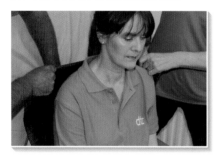

Figure 49.4 Slide the sling down to the base of the patient's back

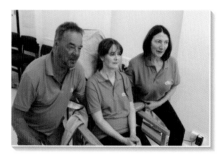

Figure 49.5 Remove the sling from the side of the chair

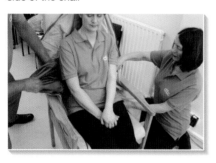

Figure 49.6 Insert the slide sheet under the patient's thigh

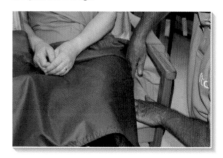

Figure 49.7 Put the leg piece between the chair and the slide sheet under the patient's thigh

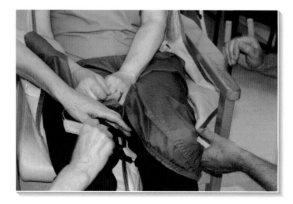

Purpose

To insert sling under the patient while in a chair.

Prior to the handling task

1   Consult any handling plans relating to this patient and check that they are clear, up-to-date and regularly reviewed.
2   If there is no written plan, ask your colleagues if they have relevant information relating to this patient.
3   Communicate with the patient and tell them what you plan to do. Ensure that they understand and obtain their consent.
4   Check that the sling is in good order. Check for rips, loose stitching, cleanliness and general condition.
5   Check that the sling has a safe working load that can take the patient.
6   If it is a disposable sling ensure that it is the patient's allocated sling and that their name is on it. Check that it has not previously got wet and that the safety label is intact.
7   If it is a reusable sling check that it has been LOLER (Lifting Operation and Lifting Equipment Regulations (1998)) checked. See Chapter 2, Legislation II. It should have been checked every six months.

During the task

1   Ask the patient to sit forward in the chair as much as they are able. Take a small roller slide and with each handler at each side of the chair they place their hands inside the slide sheet and put it behind the patient's shoulders (Figure 49.1).
2   Adopting a step stance and facing the same way as the patient, the handlers puts their inside hand inside the slide sheet and gently push the slide sheet down the side of the chair until it reaches the base of the patient's spine (Figure 49.2).
3   Take the sling and place it behind the patient's shoulders *between the chair and the slide sheet* (Figure 49.3).
4   Adopting a similar posture and stance to section 2 above, slide the sling down to the base of the patient's spine (Figure 49.4). Once it is there you can gently pull both leg pieces towards you but be careful not to pull the patient too far forward in the chair.
5   Bring the leg pieces round the side of the patient's thighs. Place your hand between the sling and the patient to ensure the patient's skin is not harmed. See Chapter 46, Insertion of sling into chair, Figure 46.2.
6   Remove the slide sheet from the side of the chair by grasping one side and pulling it through on itself. The second handler must stabilise the sling from the opposite side (Figure 49.5).
7   If the patient is unable to lift their leg(s) or lean to one side as described in Chapter 46, Insertion of sling into chair, then continue as shown further on.
8   Insert the same small roller slide sheet under the patient's thigh (Figure 49.6).
9   Once it is in place, put the leg piece between the chair and the slide sheet keeping the sling's clip or strap tucked underneath (Figure 49.7). Gently remove the slide sheet.
10   Repeat on opposite leg if necessary.
11   Check that the sling has no wrinkles or folds that can harm the patient before attaching the hoist to the sling.

After the task

1   Check that the patient has no pain and/or discomfort.
2   Check the sling is in the correct position.

50 Hoisting from bed to chair with a mobile hoist

Figure 50.1 Attach the clips or straps to the spreader bar

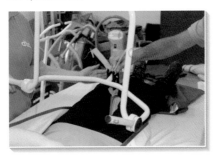

Figure 50.2 Ensure all four are attached and cross check each other's attachments

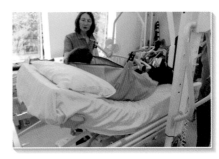

Figure 50.3 Place a small roller slide sheet under the patient's heel and bring the hoist up

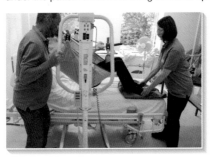

Figure 50.4 Move the patient so that their heels come off the bed while the other handler moves the hoist

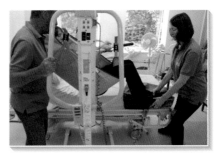

Figure 50.5 If possible, both handlers should be at either side of the hoist to move it

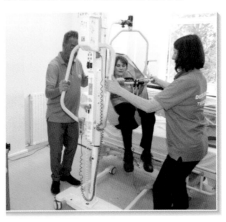

Figure 50.6 If possible place the chair diagonally between the hoist feet

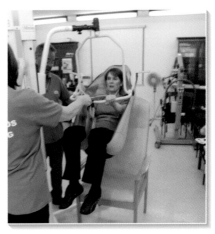

Figure 50.7 Push on the sling, the spreader bar or the patient's knees to ensure they are in the back of the chair. Use a powered spreader bar if there is one available

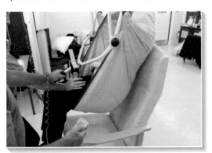

Figure 50.8 Ensure the patient is in a good position before detaching the sling

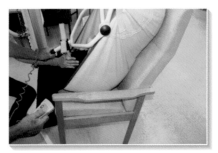

Moving and Handling Patients at a Glance. First Edition. Hamish MacGregor. © 2016 John Wiley & Sons, Ltd. Published 2016 by John Wiley & Sons, Ltd.

Purpose

To safely hoist a patient from bed to chair.

Before the technique

1   Consult any handling plans relating to this patient check that they are clear, up-to-date and regularly reviewed.

2   If there is no written plan ask your colleagues if they have relevant information relating to this patient.

3   Communicate with the patient and tell them what you plan to do. Ensure that they understand and obtain their consent.

4   Check the hoist:

- Is the safe working load of the hoist suitable for the patient?
- Has the hoist been checked/serviced in the last six months?
- Is the battery sufficient to carry out the lift?
- Where is the emergency lower?
- Where is the emergency stop?
- Does the spreader bar and the feet of the hoist move smoothly?
- Are the wheels moving smoothly?
- Do the brakes work? Note: the brakes are only used when the hoist is parked at all other times they must be off.

5   Check that the sling has a safe working load that can take the patient.

6   If it is a disposable sling ensure that it is the patient's allocated sling and that their name is on it. Check that it has not been wet and that the safety label is intact.

If it is a reusable sling check that it has been LOLER (Lifting Operation and Lifting Equipment Regulations (1998)) checked. See Chapter 2, Legislation II. It should have been checked every six months.

7   Ensure that the bed is at the correct height, that is, at the waist height of the smaller handler. Check that the sling is in good order. Check for rips, loose stitching, cleanliness and general condition.

8   Insert the sling using either of the techniques described in Chapter 44, Insertion of sling into bed; or Chapter 48, Insertion of sling into bed with two slide sheets.

During the technique

1   Sit the patient up in bed, if possible, as this makes hoisting easier for the patient and the handler.

2   The two handlers should be at either side of the bed. One handler brings the hoist in towards the patient; it should be at right angles to the bed. The second handler takes hold of the spreader bar as it moves over the patient. The spreader bar should be at chest height of the patient, not at face height.

3   The straps of the sling should be attached to the patient.

- If it is a clip type sling then attach the leg clips before the shoulder clips.
- If it is a loop type sling then the shoulder straps should be attached before the leg straps (Figures 50.1 and 50.2).

4   Cross check each other's attachments. If it is a loop type sling strap (see Chapter 43) ensure that it is attached as shown in handling plan.

- In general longer leg straps and shorter shoulder straps aid the patient into a more upright position.
- If it is a clip type sling make sure there is a firm 'click' as it is attached.

5   Place a small roller slide sheet under the patient's heels as this will reduce any friction (Figure 50.3).

6   Bring the hoist up so that there is tension on the sling and make a final check that all the loops or clips are attached.

7   Then lower the bed so that the patient is suspended in the sling. Do not lower too far as the hoist feet may get caught on the bed mechanism.

- If necessary bring the hoist up so that the patient has clearance of the bed.
- Be aware of your posture during this time and avoid stooping.

8   Move the patient so that their heels are off the bed while the other handler moves the hoist away from the bed (Figure 50.4).

- If possible, both handlers then stand at either side of the hoist and move it towards the chair (Figure 50.5).
- If possible, have the chair placed diagonally so that the patient's feet and legs do not touch the mast of the hoist (Figure 50.6).

9   Ensure that the patient is fully back in the chair by either pushing on the spreader bar, using powered spreader bar control, pushing below the patient's knees or pushing on the sling (Figures 50.7 and 50.8).

After the technique

1   Ensure that the patient is fully back in the chair and is comfortable.

2   Remove the sling as shown in Chapter 47, Removal of sling from chair.

3   Do not leave a sling under a patient unless it is specifically designed for the purpose. See Chapter 43, Types of sling – 'in-situ or all day' (see sling section for an exception to this rule).

51 Hoisting from chair to bed with a mobile hoist

Figure 51.1 Bring the hoist spreader bar in at the patient's chest height

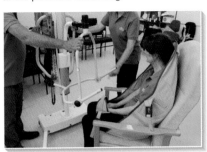

Figure 51.2 If possible, place the chair diagonally to the hoist

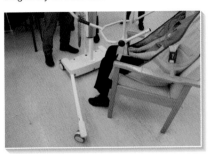

Figure 51.3 Attach the clips or loops to the spreader bar

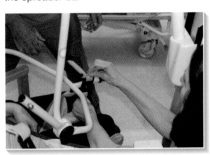

Figure 51.4 Cross check each other's clips or loops to ensure they are in place

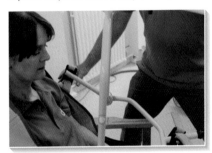

Figure 51.5 Raise the hoist until the patient is clear of the chair

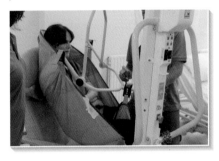

Figure 51.6 Move the hoist away from the chair

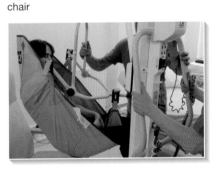

Figure 51.7 If possible, when moving the hoist stand to either side of it

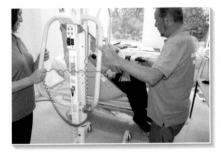

Figure 51.8 If it is a profiling bed, have it in a 'seated' position

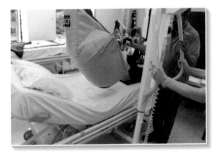

Figure 51.9 With handlers at each side of the bed, lower the patient onto the bed

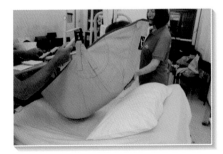

Moving and Handling Patients at a Glance. First Edition. Hamish MacGregor. © 2016 John Wiley & Sons, Ltd. Published 2016 by John Wiley & Sons, Ltd.

Purpose

To safely hoist a patient from chair to bed.

Before the technique

1 Consult any handling plans relating to this patient and check that they are clear, up-to-date and regularly reviewed.

2 If there is no written plan, ask your colleagues if they have relevant information relating to this patient.

3 Communicate with the patient and tell them what you plan to do. Ensure that they understand and obtain their consent.

4 Check the hoist:
   • Is the safe working load of the hoist suitable for the patient?
   • Has the hoist been checked/serviced in the last six months?
   • Is the battery sufficient to carry out the lift?
   • Where is the emergency lower?
   • Where is the emergency stop?
   • Does the spreader bar and the feet of the hoist move smoothly?
   • Are the wheels moving smoothly?
   • Do the brakes work? Note: the brakes are only used when the hoist is parked at all other times they must be off.

5 Check that the sling is in good order. Check for rips, loose stitching, cleanliness and general condition.

6 Check that the sling has a safe working load that can take the patient.

7 If it is a disposable sling ensure that it is the patient's allocated sling and that their name is on it. Check that it has not been wet and that the safety label is intact.

8 If it is a reusable sling check that it has been LOLER (Lifting Operation and Lifting Equipment Regulations (1998)) checked. See Chapter 2, Legislation II. It should have been checked every six months.

9 Insert the sling using either of the techniques described in Chapter 46, Insertion of sling into chair; or Chapter 49, Insertion of sling into chair with slide sheets.

During the technique

1 Bring the hoist towards the patient's chair with the spreader bar at the height of the patient's chest. One handler should guide the hoist the other with the patient guiding the spreader bar (Figure 51.1).

2 If possible have the hoist placed diagonally to the chair so that the patient's feet and legs do not touch the mast of the hoist (Figure 51.2).

3 The two handlers should be at either side of the chair and the straps of the sling should be attached to the patient.
   • If it is a clip type sling then attach the leg clips before the shoulder clips.
   • If it is a loop type sling then the shoulder straps should be attached before the leg straps (Figures 51.3 and 51.4).

4 Cross check each other's attachments.
   • If it is a loop type sling strap (see Chapter 43) ensure that it is attached as shown in handling plan.
   • In general longer leg straps and shorter shoulder straps aid the patient into a more upright position.
   • If it is a clip type sling (see Chapter 43) make sure there is a firm 'click' as it is attached.

5 Bring the hoist up so that there is tension on the sling and make a final check.

6 Bring the hoist up so that the patient has clearance of the chair. Be aware of your posture during this time and avoid stooping (Figure 51.5).

7 If possible, both handlers stand at either side of the hoist and move it towards the chair (Figures 51.6 and 51.7).

8 When the patient is above the bed ensure they are correctly placed. (If it is a profiling bed then have it in 'auto profile', that is, bed head up and knee break up so that the patient does not slide down the bed, see Figure 51.8.) Then the handlers need to aim the patient's hips into the dip. Put a small roller slide sheet at the foot of the bed to reduce the friction that may occur on the patient's heels.

9 With one handler at either side of the bed, lower the patient gently on to the bed (Figure 51.9).

After the technique

1 Ensure that the patient is comfortable and the bed is at the correct height.

2 Remove the sling as shown in Chapter 45, Removal of sling from bed.

52 Hoisting from the floor with a mobile hoist

Figure 52.1 With each handler kneeling beside the patient's hip, and with their outer foot flat on the floor, the patient should bend their knees

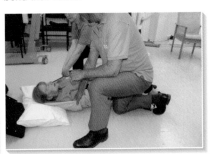

Figure 52.2 While holding the sling at the patient's shoulder, sit back on your heel to raise the patient

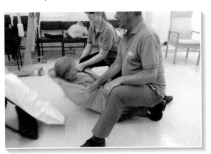

Figure 52.3 A third handler brings in an upturned chair without arms and a pillow

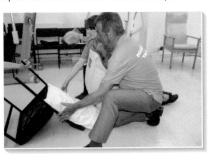

Figure 52.4 The chair and pillow are put behind the patient's back

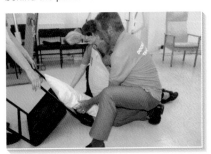

Figure 52.5 The patient is gently lowered onto the chair. The third handler stabilises the chair

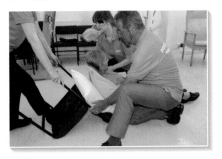

Figure 52.6 The hoist feet are opened and the hoist brought in to the side of the patient

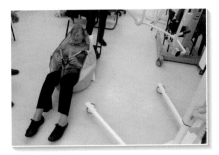

Figure 52.7 The hoist feet are placed under the chair and the patient's legs

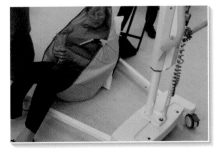

Figure 52.8 Attach the sling to the spreader bar

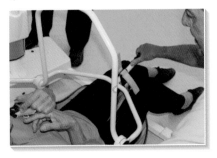

Figure 52.9 Check each other's sling connections before moving the patient

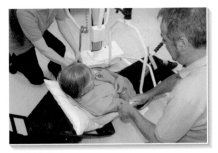

Purpose

To safely hoist a patient from the floor.

Before the technique

1   Consult any handling plans relating to this patient and check that they are clear, up-to-date and regularly reviewed.

2   If there is no written plan, ask your colleagues if they have relevant information relating to this patient.

3   Communicate with the patient and tell them what you plan to do. Ensure that they understand and obtain their consent.

4   Check the patient as shown in Chapter 22.

5   Check the hoist:

- Is the safe working load of the hoist suitable for the patient?
- Has the hoist been checked/serviced in the last six months?
- Is the battery sufficient to carry out the lift?
- Where is the emergency lower?
- Where is the emergency stop?
- Does the spreader bar and the feet of the hoist move smoothly?
- Are the wheels moving smoothly?
- Do the brakes work? Note: the brakes are only used when the hoist is parked; at all other times they must be off.

6   Check that the sling has a safe working load that can take the patient.

7   If it is a disposable sling ensure that it is the patient's allocated sling and that their name is on it. Check that it has not been wet and that the safety label is intact.

8   If it is a reusable sling check that it has been LOLER (Lifting Operation and Lifting Equipment Regulations (1998)) checked. See Chapter 2, Legislation II. It should have been checked every six months.

9   Insert the sling using the same method as described in Chapter 44, Insertion of sling into bed. This technique is identical to putting the sling in, in bed but both handlers kneel on the floor either side of the patient.

During the technique

1   If possible, sit the patient up by each handler getting either side of the patient with their inner knee aligned with the patient's hip and their outer leg foot flat on the floor, with their thigh and lower leg at 90 degrees (Figure 52.1).

2   Encourage the patient to bend their knees. The two handlers with the patient take hold of the sling at the shoulder straps with their inner hands and on the count of 'Ready, Steady, Lift', both handlers sit on their heels and the patient is sat up (Figure 52.2).

3   A third handler is behind the patient with an upturned chair that has no arms (Figure 52.3).

4   The third handler inserts the chair under the patient's pillow and the patient (Figure 52.4). If the floor is slippery then this handler may have to keep their foot on the chair to steady it.

5   The patient is gently lowered onto the pillow (Figure 52.5).

6   The patient is now in a sitting position and the hoist can be brought in from the side with the feet of the hoist inserted under the patient's knees and under the chair (Figures 52.6 and 52.7).

7   With a handler at either side of the patient, the hoist is now lowered towards the patient. One handler must take hold of the spreader bar as this is carried out.

8   The two handlers should be at either side of the patient; the straps of the sling should be attached to the patient.

- If it is a clip type sling then attach the leg clips before the shoulder clips.
- If it is a loop type sling then the shoulder straps should be attached before the leg straps (Figures 52.8 and 52.9).

9   Cross check each other's attachments.

- If it is a loop type sling strap (see Chapter 43) ensure that it is attached as shown in handling plan.
- In general longer leg straps and shorter shoulder straps aid the patient into a more upright position.
- If it is a clip type sling (see Chapter 43) make sure there is a firm 'click' as it is attached.

10   Bring the hoist up so that there is tension on the sling and make a final check.

11   Raise the patient to an appropriate height to transfer to bed and or chair.

After the technique

1   Ensure that the patient is comfortable and any observations carried out as necessary.

2   Remove the sling as shown in Chapter 45, Removal of sling from bed; or Chapter 47, Removal of sling from chair, depending if the patient has been hoisted to bed or chair.

53 Using a standing hoist

Figure 53.1 Place the sling behind patient's back

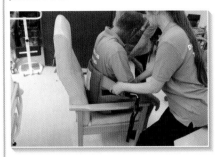

Figure 53.2 Close straps around the patient's waist

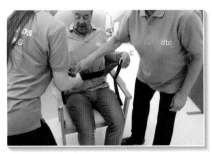

Figure 53.3 Bring in the hoist

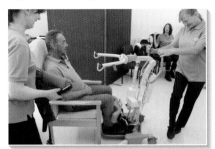

Figure 53.4 Ask the patient to place their feet flat on the footplate

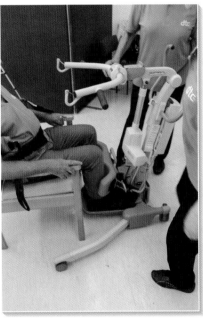

Figure 53.5 Ask the patient to hold the handgrips, and attach the strap of the sling

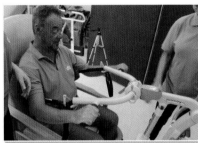

Figure 53.6 Ensure that the setting of the spreader bar is correct

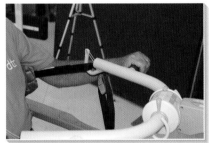

Figure 53.9 When sitting down, ensure the patient can feel the back of the chair with their legs

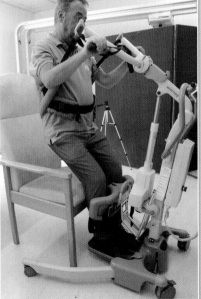

Figure 53.7 Check that there is a space between the patient's shin and the hoist

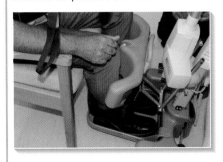

Figure 53.8 Move to the side of the hoist and, using the hand control, raise the patient

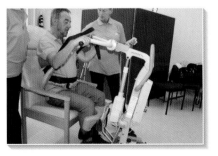

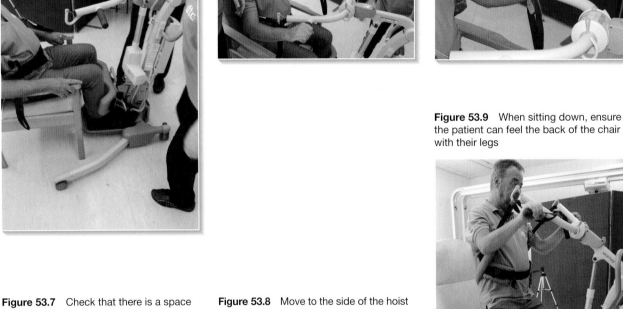

Moving and Handling Patients at a Glance. First Edition. Hamish MacGregor. © 2016 John Wiley & Sons, Ltd. Published 2016 by John Wiley & Sons, Ltd.

Purpose

To safely hoist a patient from a chair/bed/toilet/commode using a standing hoist.

Before the technique

1 Consult any handling plans relating to this patient and check that they are clear, up-to-date and regularly reviewed.

2 If there is no written plan, ask your colleagues if they have relevant information relating to this patient.

3 Communicate with the patient and tell them what you plan to do. Ensure that they understand and obtain their consent.

4 The patient must have some weight bearing ability, trunk control and the ability to cooperate and follow instructions.

5 Check the hoist:
- Is the safe working load of the hoist suitable for the patient?
- Has the hoist been checked/serviced in the last six months?
- Is the battery sufficient to carry out the lift?
- Where is the emergency lower?
- Where is the emergency stop?
- Does the sling attachment bar and the feet of the hoist move smoothly?
- Are the wheels moving smoothly?

6 Do the brakes work?

7 Checks the sling is clean, there are no rips or tears and is within the safe working load for this patient.

8 Remember all standing hoists are different and you need to ensure that you are completely familiar and competent to use the model that you are working with.

During the technique

1 Ask the patient to sit forward and put the sling behind their back (Figure 53.1). The sling needs to be placed low down the patient's back as it is important that the sling does not pull under the patient's arms. Always double the check the label on the sling for weight capacity and service check history.

2 Close the straps around the patient's waist (Figure 53.2). The straps should be fastened tightly but not so much that it causes the patient discomfort.

3 Bring in the hoist (Figure 53.3). This will usually mean opening the feet of the hoist if it has to get around the legs of a chair, for example.

4 Ask the patient to lift their feet and place them on the footplate (Figure 53.4).
- If the patient has difficulty doing this without very minimal assistance, this may indicate that a standing hoist is not the correct hoist to use as they may not have enough strength in their legs to use this piece of equipment.
- If so, carry out a re-assessment.

5 Attach the loops of the sling to the spreader bar, ensuring that they are fully in place. At the same time the patient should have their hands on the handles of the hoist and there should be a gentle tension on the straps of the sling (Figure 53.5).

6 The standing hoist illustrated has a cow horn spreader bar that can be adjusted to the height of the patient. The adjustment here is to medium (yellow) (Figure 53.6).

7 Before standing the patient up ensure that there is a gap between the patient's shins and the shin guard to allow the patient to stand easily. This must also be adjusted to ensure that it is below the patient's patella (Figure 53.7).

8 The brakes can be applied if the patient has a tendency to push the hoist away.

9 Move to the side of the hoist with the controls and stand the patient up (Figure 53.8).

10 Move the patient the *short distance* needed to bed, another chair, toilet or commode.

11 When sitting the patient down reverse the procedure, ensuring the patient can feel the back of the chair/bed/commode with their legs before they are lowered down (Figure 53.9).

After the technique

1 Remove the sling by asking the patient to sit forward.

2 Ensure that the patient is comfortable.

3 Carefully evaluate if this type of hoist is suitable for the patient and document as necessary.

54 Lateral transfer from bed to bed/trolley

Figure 54.1 Attach extension straps to the top slide sheet

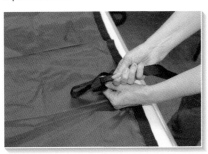

Figure 54.2 Insert PAT slide under both slide sheets, pushing into the mattress

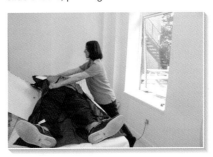

Figure 54.3 The PAT slide needs only to go under the patient to where the hole is on the edge of the mattress

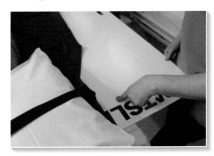

Figure 54.4 Bring in receiving bed. This should be slightly lower

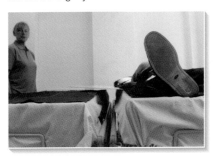

Figure 54.5 The handlers on the receiving bed take hold of the strap and adopt a walk stance position

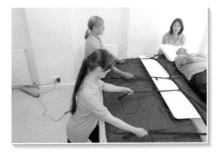

Figure 54.6 The person at the head initiates checks: brakes, height, posture

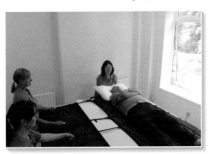

Figure 54.7 Another handler can hold the top slide sheet

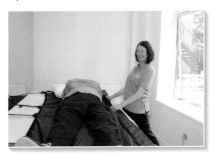

Figure 54.8 Using clear instructions, the patient is moved halfway and the handlers reposition themselves

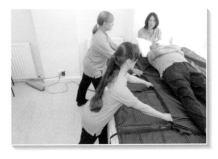

Figure 54.9 Remove handles before removing the slide sheet

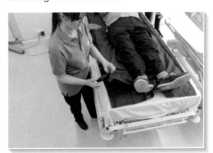

Moving and Handling Patients at a Glance. First Edition. Hamish MacGregor. © 2016 John Wiley & Sons, Ltd. Published 2016 by John Wiley & Sons, Ltd.

Purpose

To move a patient safely from one bed to another using a PAT slide.

Note: A PAT slide is a flat rectangular board usually 1525 mm × 635 mm, but this can vary. It has a smooth surface on top and a number of grip strips underneath. PAT stands for Patient Assisted Transfer and it is *not a slide* but a bridge, hence the need for slide sheets. The technique described here uses flat slide sheets with handles and extension straps. Other types of slide sheets, transfer sheets and hover devices can be used, but the principles of handling remain the same. The technique described here is a transfer from bed to bed but this can be bed to trolley or trolley to trolley.

Prior to the handling task

1 Consult any handling plans relating to this patient and check that they are clear, up-to-date and regularly reviewed.

2 If there is no written plan, ask your colleagues if they have relevant information relating to this patient.

3 Communicate with the patient and tell them what you plan to do. Ensure that they understand and obtain their consent.

4 If the patient is unconscious or has impaired conscious level then it will be necessary to have enough people to assist with the transfer.

5 Make a final check that the patient cannot do this for themselves before continuing with the task.

6 Ensure that the bed is at the correct height, that is, at waist height of the smaller handler (Figure 54.1).

During the task

1 Insert the slide sheets under the patient as described in Chapters 33–35.

2 Attach extension straps to the top slide sheet (Figure 54.1).

3 Two handlers bring in the PAT slide and insert it under the patient and both slide sheets by pushing it into the mattress. The third carer holds the slide sheets up and away from the PAT slide (Figure 54.2).

4 The PAT slide is pushed under the patient as far as the hole in the PAT slide (Figure 54.3). This is at the half way mark on the PAT slide. Some PAT slides do not have a hole so the half way mark of any PAT slide is what should be aimed for.

5 The receiving bed is brought in next to the bed. It should be slightly lower than the patient's bed (Figure 54.4).

6 The third handler passes the extension straps over the patient onto the receiving bed or trolley. Ideally there should be a third slide sheet on this bed as it will allow the patient to be easily repositioned if necessary.

7 The two handlers on the far side of the receiving bed will position themselves in a walk stance position and take hold of the straps (Figure 54.5). They must not wrap the handles around their hands.

8 The lead handler who may be a fourth handler who is by the patient's head initiates three checks as follows: (Figure 54.6).
   - Brakes? Are all the brakes on, on both beds?
   - Height? Is the receiving bed/trolley slightly lower than the patient's bed?
   - Posture? Are the two handlers adopting a walk stance position?

9 The lead carer then says, 'Ready, Steady, Slide' and the patient is moved half way across. The third handler can keep hold of the bottom slide sheet but this is not essential (Figure 54.7).

10 Once this has happened, the handlers who are pulling on the straps reposition themselves and pull the patient across the remainder of the distance (Figure 54.8).

11 Once the patient is safely on the receiving bed the other bed and the PAT slide are removed.

12 The handles are removed (Figure 54.9) and the slide sheets are removed as described in Chapter 38, Moving a patient up the bed with two flat slide sheets – 'During the task', points 7–9.

After the task

1 Check that the patient has no pain and/or discomfort and is in the correct position in the bed.

2 Put up bed rails if indicated in the handling plan and there has been an up-to-date bed rails assessment form completed.

3 Put the bed at a height that is safe for the patient.

55 Transfer from chair to bed using a transfer board

Figure 55.1 Check the board fully. Check that the rubber stickers are underneath

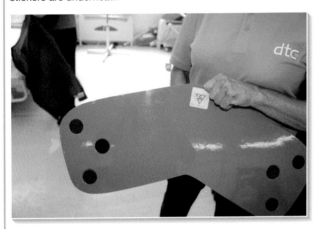

Figure 55.2 Ask the patient to lean to one side and insert one third on the board under their thigh

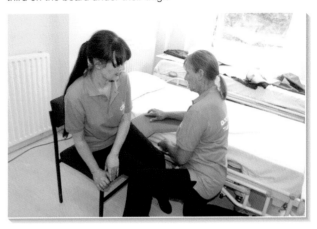

Figure 55.3 Ask the patient to put the flat of their hand on the board

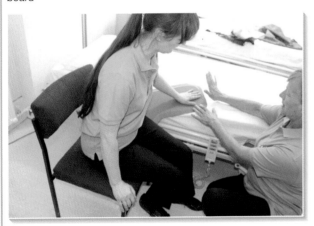

Figure 55.4 Ask the patient to transfer their body weight forward and start to move along the board

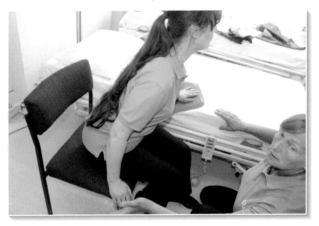

Figure 55.5 The patient continues until they are on the bed

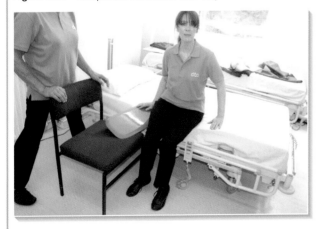

Figure 55.6 Ask the patient to lift their leg to remove the board

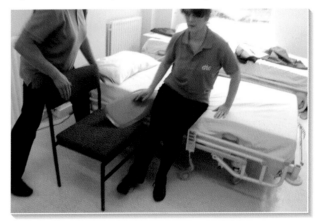

Moving and Handling Patients at a Glance. First Edition. Hamish MacGregor. © 2016 John Wiley & Sons, Ltd. Published 2016 by John Wiley & Sons, Ltd.

Purpose

To assist a patient to move from a chair to a bed while in a seated position. This can also be used from bed to chair, bed to wheelchair, chair to wheelchair and wheelchair to toilet.

The board used in the technique below is a curved board which is boomerang-shaped; these are often yellow in colour and are nicknamed banana boards. There are also straight transfer boards available.

The technique illustrates using a chair without arms, but often this is used with a wheelchair; therefore the arm of the wheelchair nearest the bed is removed to facilitate the transfer. If using a wheelchair ensure that the footplates are either removed or folded back out of the way.

Prior to the handling task

1   Consult any handling plans relating to this patient and check that they are clear, up-to-date and regularly reviewed.
2   If there is no written plan, ask your colleagues if they have relevant information relating to this patient.
3   The patient must have good upper body strength, good trunk control and an ability to understand and follow instructions to carry out this procedure.
4   Communicate with the patient and tell them what you plan to do. Ensure that they understand and obtain their consent.
5   Check that the patient has suitable clothing as bare skin will not slide on the board and skin can be damaged.
6   Check that the transfer board is clean and in good condition with no damage to the surface or edges. Any rubber adhesion dots or strips should be intact (Figure 55.1).

7   It is not advisable to use a slide sheet to help the patient slide across as there is little control over the movement and the patient could fall.

During the task

1   Get the chair as close to the bed as possible. The chair should be slightly higher or level with the bed. Get down to the side of the patient's chair. The patient must be able to put their feet firmly on the floor and must be wearing suitable footwear. This technique can also be used for patients with lower limb amputations. Be careful to ensure that you have a good posture.
2   Ask the patient to lean to one side, away from the bed, so that they are transferring to the board, and insert the transfer board under the patient's buttock. About one third of the board is sufficient (Figure 55.2).
3   Ask the patient to put their hand towards the edge of the board ensuring that their fingers do not go under the board as they may become trapped as they slide across the board (Figure 55.3).
4   Patient transfers their body weight and slides across to the centre of the board (Figures 55.4 and 55.5).
5   The patient continues across the board until they reach the bed. Ask the patient to lift their leg nearest the chair so that the board can be removed (Figure 55.6).

After the task

1   Check that the patient has no pain and/or discomfort.
2   Check that they are clear how to carry out this task again and document any findings.

56 Assisting a patient to use a rota-stand: one handler

Figure 56.1 Check whether the patient can lift their hips off the bed

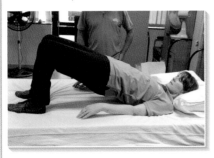

Figure 56.2 Bring in the rota-stand to the patient

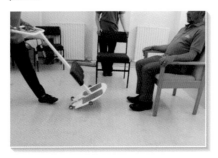

Figure 56.3 Ask the patient to put their foot on to the footplate

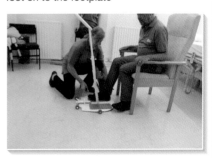

Figure 56.4 Ensure that both feet are placed centrally on the footplate

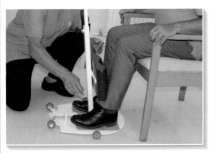

Figure 56.5 Ensure there is a gap between the rota stand and the patient's shin

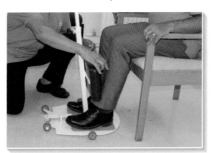

Figure 56.6 Encourage the patient to move forward on the chair

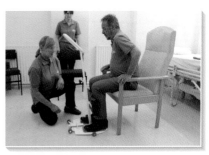

Figure 56.7 Ask the patient to hold the handle

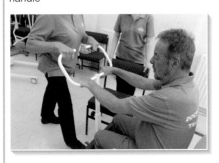

Figure 56.8 With your foot on the brake, ask the patient to stand

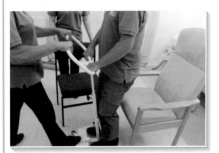

Figure 56.9 Adopting a good posture, turn the rota stand

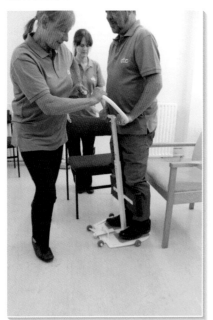

Figure 56.10 With your foot on the brake, ask the patient to sit. Ensure they can feel the back of the chair

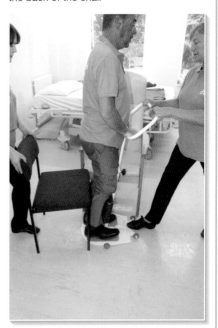

Moving and Handling Patients at a Glance. First Edition. Hamish MacGregor. © 2016 John Wiley & Sons, Ltd. Published 2016 by John Wiley & Sons, Ltd.

Purpose

To assist a patient to move from bed to chair. This technique can also be used for a transfer from chair to chair, chair to commode, wheelchair to toilet, etc.

Assessment

To assess whether the patient can safely use this piece of equipment. The assessment will check if the patient can:

• Demonstrate some active hip extension, for example, can bridge on bed (Figure 56.1).

• Demonstrate sitting balance. See Chapter 14, Assessing the patient before standing from the chair – 'During the assessment', point 9, for one method of testing this.

• Place and maintain their aligned feet on the footplate with the assistance of one handler.

• Place their hands on hand grips with assistance of one handler.

• Move from the back to the front of chair to standing independently or with the assistance of one handler (this handler cannot also counterbalance the rota-stand).

• Stand for sufficient time to allow the rota-stand to be turned through 90 degrees and wait to be instructed before sitting.

• Sit from standing.

• Follow instructions adequately.

Prior to the handling task

1 Consult any handling plans relating to this patient. Check that they are clear, up-to-date and regularly reviewed.

2 If there is no written plan, ask your colleagues if they have relevant information relating to this patient.

3 Communicate with the patient and tell them what you plan to do. Ensure that they understand and obtain their consent.

4 The chair or commode to which the patient is being transferred must be placed at right angles to the chair that the patient is sitting on.

5 *Check that it is safe for one handler to carry out this task with the patient. If in any doubt get a second handler.*

During the task

1 Bring the rota-stand to the patient (Figure 56.2).

2 Ask the patient to put their foot on the rota-stand (Figure 56.3).

3 Ensure that both the patient's feet are located centrally on the footplate (Figure 56.4).

4 There should be a gap of approximately 3 cm between the patient's shin and the padded shin guard (Figure 56.5). Some rota-stands have an adjustable shin guard, if so always ensure that it is below the knee.

5 Encourage the patient to move forward in the chair (Figure 56.6).

6 Ask the patient to put both hands onto the rota-stand or one hand on the rota-stand and one on the arm of the chair (Figure 56.7).

7 The first handler's foot is put firmly on the brake and acting as a counterbalance by holding the top of the rota-stand handle. The patient should bring themselves forward to keep their weight over the centre footplate, that is, not leaning back. Then the patient brings themselves into a standing position (Figure 56.8).

8 The handler turns the rota-stand ensuring that they adopt a good posture and minimise twisting (Figure 56.9).

9 The patient is rotated towards the receiving chair/commode.

10 A second handler may have to adjust the position of the receiving chair so that the back of the patient's knees are touching it.

11 With the first handler with their foot firmly on the brake of the rota-stand and their weight acting as a counterbalance, the patient sits down in the chair. Ask the patient to reach with one arm down onto the chair as this will encourage natural body movement as they sit down (Figure 56.10).

After the task

1 Check that the patient has no pain and/or discomfort.

2 Ensure that the patient is in the best functional position.

57 Assisting a patient to use a rota-stand: two handlers

Figure 57.1 With one handler's foot on the brake, the second handler encourages the patient to sit forward

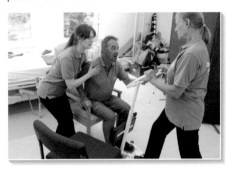

Figure 57.2 With the patient's hand on the handle of the rota-stand, the handler guides the patient forward

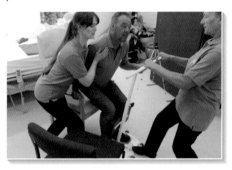

Figure 57.3 Once the patient is stable, the rota-stand can be turned. A hand on the patient's back may give reassurance

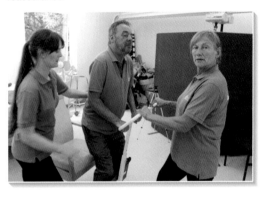

Figure 57.4 The second handler can stabilise the chair

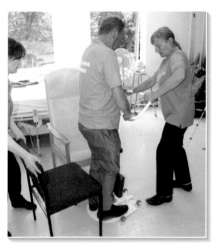

Figure 57.5 The second handler can put their hand between the patient's shoulder blades

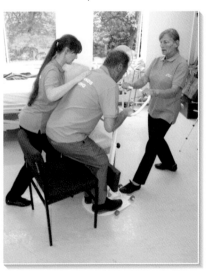

Figure 57.6 Ensure the patient is sitting fully back in the chair

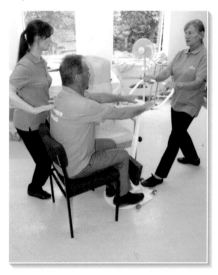

Purpose

To assist a patient to move from bed to chair. This technique can also be used for a transfer from chair to chair, chair to commode, wheelchair to toilet, etc.

Assessment

To assess whether the patient can safely use this piece of equipment. The assessment will check if the patient can:

• Demonstrate some active hip extension, for example, can bridge on bed (see Figure 56.1 in Chapter 56).
• Demonstrate sitting balance. See Chapter 14, Assessing the patient before standing up from the chair – 'During the assessment', point 9, for one method of testing this.
• Place and maintain their aligned feet on the footplate with the assistance of one handler.
• Place their hands on hand grips with the assistance of one handler.
• Move from the back to the front of the chair to standing independently or with the assistance of one handler (this handler cannot also counterbalance the rota-stand).
• Stand for sufficient time to allow the rota-stand to be turned through 90 degrees and wait to be instructed before sitting.
• Sit from standing.
• Follow instructions adequately.

Prior to the handling task

1 Consult any handling plans relating to this patient. Check that they are clear, up-to-date and regularly reviewed.
2 If there is no written plan ask your colleagues if they have relevant information relating to this patient.
3 Communicate with the patient and tell them what you plan to do. Ensure that they understand and obtain their consent.
4 The chair or commode to which the patient is being transferred must be placed at right angles to the chair that the patient is sitting on.

During the task

1 Follow points 1–7 in Chapter 56, Assisting a patient to use a rota-stand: one handler.
2 Handler one has their foot firmly on the brake of the rota-stand. The second handler adopts a walk stance position and on the command of 'Ready, Steady, Stand', (or other commands agreed with the patient) assists the patient to stand up (Figure 57.1). See Chapter 16, Standing a patient up from a chair with one handler, for more information.
3 When the patient is assisted to stand they must take the initiative with the second handler guiding (Figure 57.2).
4 Once the patient is standing and is stable, the first handler begins to rotate the stand around. The second handler may keep their hand on the patient's back for reassurance (Figure 57.3).
5 The patient should be rotated round as in point 9 in Chapter 56.
6 When the patient can feel the back of the receiving chair with the back of their legs, they can be encouraged to sit down. Ask the patient to reach with one arm down onto the chair as this will encourage natural body movement as they sit down. The second handler may have to adjust the position of the receiving chair at this point. The first handler has their foot on the rota-stand brake. The second handler may stabilise the chair (Figure 57.4).
7 Alternatively, as the patient sits down the second handler can place their hand between the patient's shoulder blades (Figure 57.5). See Chapter 18, Seating a patient, for more information.
8 Ensure that the patient is sitting fully back in their chair (Figure 57.6).

After the assessment

1 Check that the patient has no pain and/or discomfort.
2 Ensure that the patient is in the best functional position.

58 Use of standing and raising aids (non-mechanical)

Figure 58.1 Check that patient can lift their hips off the bed

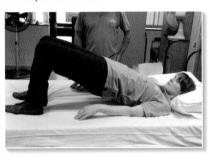

Figure 58.2 Bring the Stedy in towards the patient and ask them to put their feet on the footplate

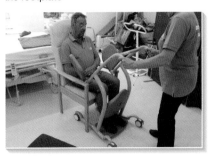

Figure 58.3 Put the brakes on

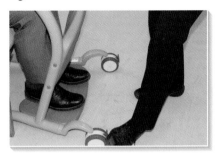

Figure 58.4 Ask the patient to stand up

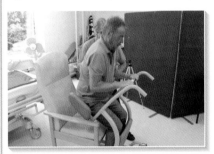

Figure 58.5 When the patient is standing, bring the seat paddles down

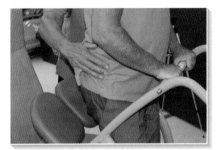

Figure 58.6 Release the brakes and move the patient

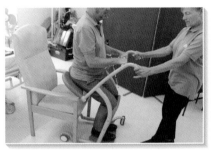

Figure 58.7 Ask the patient to stand and flip back the seat paddles

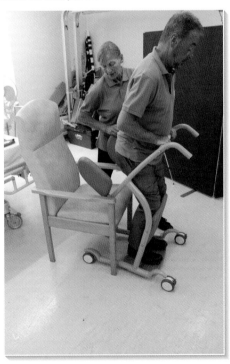

Figure 58.8 Ask the patient to sit fully back in the chair

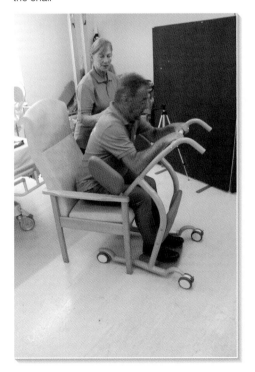

Moving and Handling Patients at a Glance. First Edition. Hamish MacGregor. © 2016 John Wiley & Sons, Ltd. Published 2016 by John Wiley & Sons, Ltd.

There are a number of examples of this type of equipment on the market, such as the Helping Hand Cricket 1, Cricket 2, the Arjo Stedy (used here) and the Sara Stedy.

This type of equipment often bridges the gap between a standing hoist (Chapter 53), a rota-stand (Chapters 56 and 57) and a wheelchair.

Purpose

To assist the patient to move from the bed to a chair. This technique can also be used to transfer from one chair to another chair, a chair to a commode, or a wheelchair to a toilet, etc.

Assessment

To assess whether the patient can safely use this piece of equipment. The assessment will check if the patient can:

• Demonstrate some active hip extension, for example, can bridge on the bed (Figure 58.1).

• Demonstrate sitting balance. See Chapter 14, Assessing the patient before standing up from the chair – 'During the assessment', point 9, for one method of testing this.

• Place and maintain their aligned feet on the footplate with the assistance of one handler.

• Place their hands on bar with the assistance of one handler.

• Move from the back to the front of the chair to standing independently or with the assistance of one handler.

• Move from sitting to standing.

• Follow instructions adequately.

Prior to the handling task

1   Consult any handling plans relating to this patient. Check that they are clear, up-to-date and regularly reviewed.

2   If there is no written plan, ask your colleagues if they have relevant information relating to this patient.

3   Communicate with the patient and tell them what you plan to do. Ensure that they understand and obtain their consent.

4   *Check that this is safe for one handler to carry out this task with the patient. If in any doubt get a second handler.*

During the handling task

1   Bring the Stedy in towards the patient. This must come directly in front of the patient. Some other models such as the Sara Stedy have adjustable feet that make it easier to get in front of the chair (Figure 58.2).

2   Ask the patient to move forward in the chair and put their feet on the footplate.

• Feet must be flat on the footplate with the hips and knees at 90 degrees.

• Remember if the patient is unable to do this then this is not the correct equipment for them to use.

• Put the brakes on to prevent the patient from pushing the Stedy away (Figure 58.3).

• Ensure that there is a space between the patient's shins and the shin plate of the Stedy.

3   Ask the patient to pull themselves forward by pulling on the bar. Putting your hand behind the patient's back may give them reassurance and encourage them to fully participate in the manoeuvre (Figure 58.4).

4   If the patient needs more assistance then cross your hand round the patient's back and place your hand on the iliac crest. See Chapter 16, Standing a patient up from the chair with one handler, for more detailed information.

5   When the patient is fully into standing, bring the seat paddles down and encourage the patient to sit down. Give the patient some time to recover before you move to the next stage of the manoeuvre (Figure 58.5).

6   When the patient is ready, release the brakes and slowly move the patient to a wheelchair, other chair, bed, commode, or toilet as appropriate (Figure 58.6).

7   To sit the patient down, reverse the procedure.

8   The Stedy is placed over the chair, the chair and the brakes are engaged. Move to the side and ask the patient to stand up. You may need to give assistance as described previously depending on the patient's abilities. Once the patient is standing, lift one seat paddle up and then the other.

• Ensure that you do not overstretch as you carry this out.

• Ensure that you are continually explaining to the patient what you are doing (Figure 58.7).

9   Encourage the patient to sit back in the chair, placing their arms on the back of the chair one at a time. To facilitate this, place your hand at the centre of the patient's back between the shoulder blades (Figure 58.8). See Chapter 18, Seating a patient, for more detailed information.

10   When the patient is comfortable, remove the Stedy.

After the task

1   Check that the patient has no pain and/or discomfort.

2   Ensure that the patient is in the best functional position.

59 Use of equipment for bariatric patients

Figure 59.1 Examples of bariatric beds

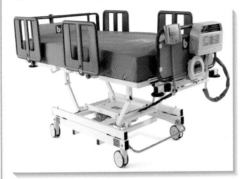

(a) Aurum bariatric bed

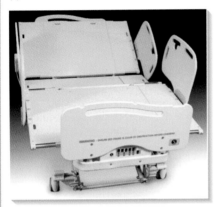

(b) Extendable bariatric bed

Figure 59.2 Examples of bariatric chairs

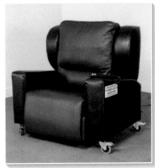

(a) Riser recliner chair

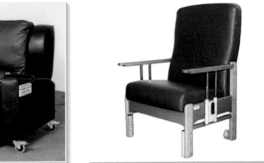

(b) Adjustable height static chair
with drop down arms

Figure 59.3 Examples of commodes

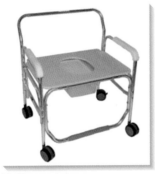

(a) Shower chair

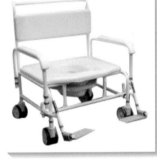

(b) 53st bariatric commode

Figure 59.4 Toilet support and surround

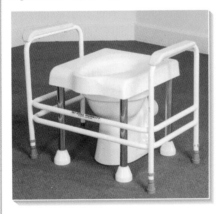

Figure 59.5 Mobile bariatric hoist

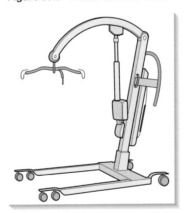

Figure 59.6 Gantry hoist with twin motors

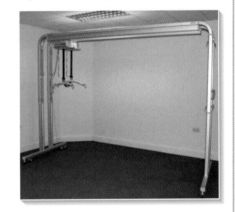

Figure 59.7 Bariatric sling

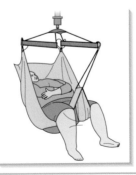

Figure 59.8 Lift pants

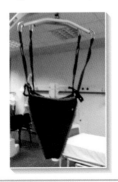

*Figures 59.1a, 59.2b, 59.3a and 59.6
reproduced with permission of
Benmor Medical:
www.benmormedical.co.uk*

*Figures 59.1b, 59.2a, 59.3b and 59.4
reproduced with permission of
1st Call Mobility:
http://www.1stcallmobility.co.uk*

Purpose

To introduce equipment that might be of use when caring for a bariatric patient. The selection of the correct equipment is always dependent on a suitable and sufficient moving and handling assessment.

Definition

The origin of the word bariatric comes from the Greek words *barys* meaning heavy and *baros* meaning weight. Definitions of who can be described as bariatric vary (often over 159 kg/25 stone) but often it is when equipment such as beds, chairs and moving and handling aids have a safe working load (SWL) that is less than the patient's weight. It is for this reason that a patient's weight needs to be obtained as soon as possible after accessing a health or social care service. Often it is the size and shape of a patient that will determine the choice of equipment rather than their weight.

The management of the bariatric patient can be complex and this chapter only introduces the topic. The choice of equipment is going to look at two groups of patient, the mobile and the dependent patient.

The mobile patient

The mobile patient may need equipment due to their weight, size or shape. It is important to realise that just because a patient is large they may not be immobile. A comprehensive assessment will determine the patient's mobility and focus on maintaining the patient's independence.

Equipment to consider

Bed

A modern standard hospital profiling bed often has an SWL of 250 kg/39 stone, so often having an alternative bed is not necessary. Be aware an SWL does not mean that the bed will take a patient of that weight, as one has to allow for the weight of equipment attached to the bed, for example, a power unit of low air loss mattress or oxygen cylinder. There is a range of bariatric beds available to purchase or hire. These can have expandable sides that vary from 36″ to 42″ to 48″ widths. Be aware that if the bed is at the full width then it may be too difficult to work with the patient as the posture of the handler will be severely compromised. See examples of these beds in Figure 59.1. These beds can have an SWL of up to 450 kg/70 stone. Other features of such beds can be:

- The ability to go down lower to the floor, which will allow shorter patients to maintain their mobility.
- Integral weighing scales.
- Egress handles to assist the patient to get in and out of the bed.
- A choice of mattresses both static and dynamic; the important thing here is that the mattress has sufficient pressure relieving properties for the weight of that patient.

Chairs

Many chairs have quite low SWL, or there is no reliable information available. There is a huge range of static chairs and riser recliner chairs that take weights up to 320 kg/50 stone. These chairs come in a range of seat widths and depths. The static chairs can be height adjustable and have drop-down arms which can allow for easier transfer into bed. Examples of these chairs are shown in Figure 59.2.

Commodes and shower chairs

Like chairs, these come in different weight capacities and widths with some commodes doubling as shower chairs. Examples of these are shown in Figure 59.3.

Toilet supports and surrounds

These can be placed over and around the toilet to increase the weight limit of the toilet, and also to give a secure handle for the patient to push themselves up from the toilet. These are pictured in Figure 59.4.

Walking aids

A bariatric patient may need a heavy duty walking frame. These are available for up to 320 kg/50 stone.

The dependent patient

All of the equipment described here may be needed. Additionally other equipment may have to be sourced.

Equipment to consider

Hoists

There are mobile hoists that have a SWL of 320 kg/50 stone (Figure 59.5) and gantry hoists (Figure 59.6) that have a maximum user weight of 500 kg/78 stone.

Slings

Slings of a suitable size and shape will have to be sourced that are compatible with the hoist (Figure 59.7). There are also specialist slings such as 'Lift Pants' (Figure 59.8) that can be placed around the patient and uses the hoist to lift the patient into a standing position. This will allow the hoist to take the patient's weight while giving the handlers the opportunity to assist the patient to stand.

Mattresses

In addition to looking at the pressure relieving qualities of the mattress, a turning mattress may be needed for the more dependent patient. This will not only help maintain the patient's skin integrity, but it will also make it easier for the handlers to move the patient in bed.

Slide sheets

Extra wide slide sheets may be necessary to move the patient and use of repositioning sheets may also reduce the amount of patient handling which can reduce staff injury and increase patient comfort and dignity.

Note: This is not a comprehensive list, but gives examples of equipment commonly used.

60 Kneeling and working at floor level

Figure 60.1   Jolly back chair

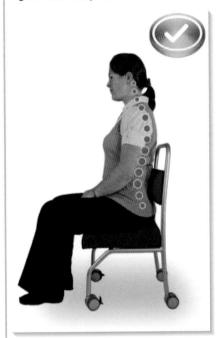

Figure 60.2   Use of kneeling pads

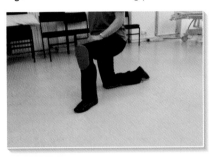

Figure 60.3   Using a pillow to improve posture

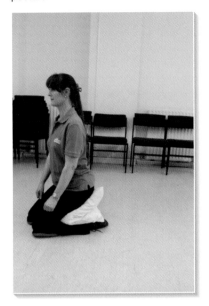

Figure 60.5   Ergokneeler

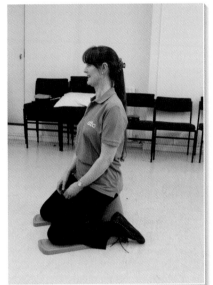

Figure 60.8   Sitting forward

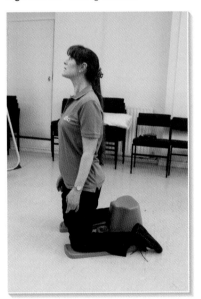

Figure 60.4   Norwich kneeling stool

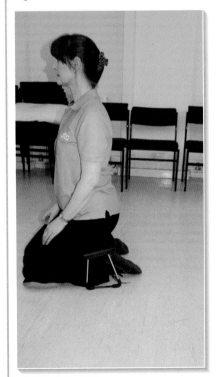

Figure 60.6   Full kneeling

Figure 60.7   Half kneeling

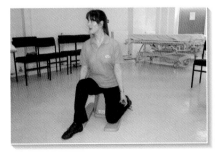

Figure 60.9   Using as a stool

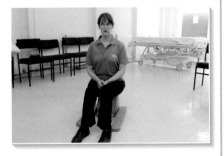

Purpose

To raise awareness of the potential problems with kneeling and working at a low level. There are many situations in which health care and social care workers have to kneel for prolonged periods. These include leg ulcer dressings in the community, working with children and dressing lower limbs of patients when they are in a chair.

Prior to any procedure involving kneeling or working at floor level

1   Look at alternatives that may be available that might be better for posture.

2   See what equipment there is around that may be available that could reduce pressure on your knees.

3   Think how it might be possible to split the kneeling task into smaller component parts that would allow periods to change posture.

4   Can the kneeling task be divided between more members of staff therefore reducing the risk of cumulative injury to one person?

During the task

It is often something simple like a low stool, particularly when working with children, that can be a simple risk-reducing measure. This will prevent the need to kneel and therefore eliminate many of the problems. These can be simple stools through to the 'Jolly back chair' seen in Figure 60.1. The Jolly back chair can help maintain good posture and is available in three different sizes depending on the child age range and the height of the adult.

Often it is not possible to avoid kneeling. When kneeling, it is important not only to think of reducing strain to your back, but also hips, knees, ankles and feet.

Here are some options that may help.

Kneeling pads

These can be worn under trousers if necessary and can act as a cushion for the knees; this is particularly important when one has to kneel on a hard surface (Figure 60.2).

It is very easy to adopt a poor posture when you are kneeling. This manifests itself by adopting a C-shaped spine with the knees fully flexed. The simplest solution to this is to put a pillow or cushion behind the knees. This has the effect of taking the knees out of full flexion thereby reducing the tendency to slump (Figure 60.3).

Kneeling stools

There are particular pieces of equipment such as the Norwich kneeling stool that is designed to carry out the above functions. This is a light portable stool that folds flat and is wipe clean. When the person kneels down they place the stool under their hips and sit down (Figure 60.4).

A more sophisticated piece of equipment is the Ergokneeler. This is a lightweight foam stool made of wipe clean material. This is multifunctional as it allows the person to change their posture frequently when they are kneeling. This is particularly important when there is prolonged kneeling.

This piece of equipment has built in kneeling pads, therefore direct pressure on the knees can be reduced. These pads are an integral part of the equipment and can be adjusted in length (Figure 60.5).

Various postures that can be adopted with an ergokneeler

Full kneeling

As there is an integral stool this allows for a good posture to be adopted: the knees are not fully flexed and the ankle are not fully stretched (Figure 60.6).

Half kneeling

This allows for a change in posture while still adopting a good posture with the knee supported on a padded surface and the opposite foot flat on the floor (Figure 60.7).

Sitting forward

This allows for the person to sit fully forward with both knees supported on a cushioned surface (Figure 60.8).

Using as a stool

The person can change posture and use the piece of equipment as a low stool (Figure 60.9).

In addition to all of this it is important that when working at a low level that you try and bring things you are working with up from the floor and at a height that allows you to adopt a better posture. If you are carrying out a procedure at a low level, ensure that the equipment you need is at hand as it is easy to bend and twist at the same time, increasing the possible cumulative injury to your back. Planning the activity before you start a procedure is vital, as stretching to reach a piece of equipment when you are kneeling or sitting puts a great strain on the lower back and can contribute to cumulative injury.

Important: **None of the equipment described above will help reduce muscle-skeletal injury unless you are aware of your posture.**

Case study 1: Assessing a bariatric patient

John is a 56-year-old man who has been admitted to the Medical Admissions Unit with pain in his right leg which means that he is unable to weight bear. He is very large, but neither he nor his family has any idea of his current weight. He tells the staff that he weighed 40 stone (254 kg) about 9 months ago.

He has been in bed at home for the past week and his condition has not improved. He now has some breathing problems and there is a query about a chest infection.

He is a pleasant man who has some understanding of his medical condition, but is naturally very anxious.

The immediate moving and handling issues are to get an accurate weight to ensure that he is on the correct bed or chair that will take his weight. In addition this will allow the correct dosage of any medication he needs to be prescribed.

The potential risks are identified in Table CS1. Please read this through now before moving on. More information on the moving and handling risk assessment process is provided in Chapter 7.

All the equipment mentioned below can be hired as well as bought. There are a number of specialist bariatric equipment specialists who will hire equipment and often deliver within four hours.

Some options for weighing John

- Obtain a bariatric bed with integral weighing scales. This will necessitate transferring him onto another bed.
- Obtain bed shoe scales which will allow him to be weighed in his current bed. These can be slid under the wheels of the existing bed and allow the patient to be weighed.
- Hoist him off the bed with a bariatric hoist with integral weighing scales. There are mobile hoists with weighing scales that can weigh up to 320 kg/50 stone. See Chapter 59 for an example of this.

Obtaining the correct bed

Hospital beds vary in their capacity. In this case it is very likely that John will need a specialist bariatric bed. Remember a bed's safe working load is different from maximum patient weight as there needs to be an allowance given for equipment that is attached to the bed.

As well as safe working load, there needs to be thought given to the patient's girth. This could mean that a bed was needed that had expandable sides for patient comfort. See Chapter 59 for an example of this.

Consideration would need to be given to the height of the bed, as to aid mobilisation a bed that will come down lower may allow the patient to get in and out of bed more easily. If John had been of short stature he may have needed a bed that could be lowered nearer to the floor. Before obtaining a bed, check the lowest height of the base from the floor, taking into account the mattress that will be used on the bed.

Consider if it will be advantageous to have a bed with an integral weighing scale. This will allow the patient's weight to be monitored throughout their hospital stay.

Obtaining the correct mattress

A standard hospital mattress will have a maximum patient weight. In John's case he will probably need a specialist mattress that would have enough pressure-relieving properties to ensure that any tissue viability issues are minimised.

There are static and dynamic mattresses available. John would benefit from a dynamic mattress with a turning facility that could be programmed to turn at specific time intervals.

Other equipment

As well as beds and mattresses, other equipment may need to be sourced.

Hoists and slings: As well as mobile hoists there are gantry hoists that can be placed over the bed and allow easier transfer from bed to chair. John would benefit from a gantry hoist — as well as making hoisting easier for him and the staff, it would also be easier to use lift pants (see Chapter 59 for an example). This would make it easier during early mobilisation which would be beneficial for an effective discharge.

Chairs, commodes, toilet surrounds and walking frames are all examples of equipment that will need an increased safe working load for John to be able to use safely.

Staff training and competence

Staff will often need additional moving and handling training to ensure they are competent in managing a larger patient. As this is a skill that may not be used on a regular basis, thought needs to be given to how staff maintain their competence. It is for this reason that if the patient is in a specialist unit, care can be more effectively delivered.

Dignity issues

The larger patient needs to be treated with the utmost dignity and respect and it can be easy to fall into the trap of judging someone who weighs more than you do. The provision of well-trained staff with access to the correct equipment will always improve patient dignity. If there is a lack of equipment or staff who do not know how to use it then there are often too many staff dealing with the patient at the same time.

Discharge

A clear discharge plan is necessary to ensure there is the right equipment (with well-trained care staff if necessary) in place when the patient goes home.

Moving and Handling Patients at a Glance. First Edition. Hamish MacGregor. © 2016 John Wiley & Sons, Ltd. Published 2016 by John Wiley & Sons, Ltd.

Table CS1 The component parts in a moving and handling risk assessment (see Chapter 7 for more details)

The task

Factors that may need to be considered	Risk-reducing measures	Equipment issues
• Can you apply the key safe principles of handling? (see Chapter 5)	Ensure staff are trained, competent and posturally aware	
• Be aware of static postures (see Chapter 4)	Ensure staff are trained, competent and posturally aware	
• Can you avoid twisting?	Ensure staff are trained, competent and posturally aware	
• Do you need to carry over a long distance?	Not applicable	
• Are there unpredictable movements of loads?	Not applicable	
• Does this involve repetitive handling?	This should not be an issue if staff are suitably trained	
• Are there sufficient breaks factored into the task?	Not applicable	

Individual capability

Factors that may need to be considered	Risk-reducing measures	Equipment issues
• Require a certain level of fitness?	Are staff encouraged to keep themselves fit?	
• Present a risk to those who have pre-existing health problems?	Ensure that no staff with a current or pre-existing musculoskeletal problem works with the patient on a regular basis	If there is suitable and sufficient equipment this should not be a problem
• Constitute a hazard to those who are pregnant?	Pregnant staff should have had a pregnancy risk assessment. See HSE flow chart: www.hse.gov.uk/mothers/docs/pregnant-workers-flow-chart.pdf	
• Require specialised training?	Additional training may be required for some staff not familiar or experienced in working with a patient with these specific handling needs	Additional training on equipment may be required
• Require a certain level of knowledge, skills and competency?	Ensure staff are trained, competent and posturally aware	
• Become more risky at certain times of the day?	Staff who work 'long days' should be aware of the potential increased risk at the end of their working day	

The load

Factors that may need to be considered	Risk-reducing measures	Equipment issues
• Heavy?	*See person section below*	
• Bulky?		
• Difficult to grasp?		
• Unstable or have an uneven weight distribution?		
• Potentially harmful, for example, hot		

Person factors

Factors that may need to be considered	Risk-reducing measures	Equipment issues
• The patient has been identified as large and has handling needs to be addressed	Ensure there are enough staff who are skilled and competent at managing a patient with these handling needs	Suitable and sufficient equipment needs to be sourced as soon as possible
• Medical conditions that will affect handling	The management of his inability to weight bear and his chest infection needs to be addressed by the multidisciplinary team	
• Level of understanding?	Not applicable	
• Level of cooperation?	Not applicable	
• Conscious level?	Not applicable	
• Pain?	Patient's pain needs to be monitored and controlled. Adequate pain control must be given before any moving and handling is carried out	
• Attachments, i/v lines, catheters, drains?	Additional member of staff may be needed to look after these when the patient is moved	

The environment

Factors that may need to be considered	Risk-reducing measures	Equipment issues
• Is there enough space?	Removing any unnecessary equipment from the patient area.	Bariatric equipment by its nature is large and requires additional space
• Type of flooring?	Not applicable in hospital but may have to be addressed before the patient is discharged home.	
• Are there stairs to be negotiated?	Not applicable in hospital but may have to be addressed before the patient is discharged home	
• Is there a good ergonomic layout?	Plan any move ahead of time to maximise the use of the available space. Before being discharged an Occupational Therapist will need to carry out a home visit to assess layout at home	
• Are there obstacles in the way?	Remove as necessary before any move is carried out	
• Is the temperature conducive to the work being carried out?	Staff to keep themselves well hydrated as the patient may prefer a warmer room temperature	
• Is there sufficient lighting?	Ensure there is good lighting	

Equipment

Factors that may need to be considered	Risk-reducing measures	Equipment issues
• Is it appropriate for the task?	Ensure all necessary equipment is sourced	Think of all the equipment that may be needed, for example: bed, chair, hoist, sling, commode, walking frame, etc.
• Has the safe working load been identified?	Obtaining an accurate weight of the patient and matching that with the equipment used	
• Is it in good working order and free from damage?	Having a planned maintenance programme. Staff made aware of need to check equipment before it is used	
• Has it been serviced/checked in accordance with legal requirements, for example, LOLER? (see Chapter 2)	Ensure LOLER checks are up-to-date and staff aware of their responsibility to check the equipment	
• Do the staff require any special training to operate the equipment?	Additional training on equipment may be required	

Other influencing factors

Factors that may need to be considered	Risk-reducing measures	Equipment issues
• Levels of stress or other psychosocial factors	Are there policies in place to manage staff who may be experiencing stress?	
• Poor staffing levels supplemented by high numbers of agency staff.	If this is an ongoing issue are there robust systems in place to record, monitor and escalate staffing problems to senior management	
• Pressures of work or at home	Staff feel comfortable to discuss these issues with manager	
• Organisational policies	Ensure there is appropriate policy and protocols for the management of the bariatric patient. This will include the access to suitable equipment in a timely manner	

Case study 2: Managing leg ulcer dressings in the community (kneeling)

> Mary is an 87-year-old woman who lives at home with her 90-year-old husband. He is her main carer and although he is physically frail he would rather care for her than have the home care service involved.
>
> Mary has arthritis which restricts her mobility and causes her a lot of pain. She is housebound and has a riser recliner beside the bed, where she spends most of the day. She still likes to get out of bed early and her husband manages to transfer her from bed to chair in the morning and back in the evening.
>
> Her main problem is a leg ulcer that she has dressed weekly by the community nurse. This involves the nurse soaking off the dressing in a bucket of water, then redressing the wound and applying the pressure bandages.
>
> The room is small and cluttered and the community nurses all complain of backache after attending to Mary.

The potential risks are identified in Table CS2. Please read this through now before moving on. More information on the moving and handling risk assessment process is provided in Chapter 7. The information on kneeling options is in Chapter 60 and is referred to below.

Soaking-off the dressing in a bucket of water

This was being filled in the bath then carried through to the bedroom.

There are a number of handling issues here, such as lifting a heavy bucket of water out of the bath and then carrying it. This was made simpler by having the bucket on a small low trolley, a hose attached to the tap, and the bucket filled and then wheeled though to Mary. It was also found that the bucket did not need to be filled so full. This reduces the handling risk, but does not eliminate it.

The other alternatives here would be that the dressing was soaked off in the bath or shower, but as Mary was only washed in bed this was not an option.

Other load handling issues

The community nurse could use a back pack which had wheels to carry her equipment to patients' houses.

Environmental issues

The room is small and cluttered, which made it difficult for the nurses to get into a safe posture when attending to Mary's leg ulcer dressing. The ideal solution would be to move to a larger room, but Mary and her husband did not find this acceptable. It was agreed to clear some small pieces of furniture out of the room, remove the loose rugs and therefore have a clear way from the bathroom to the bedroom and around Mary. If the above agreement had not been reached, it may have been necessary to arrange transport to bring Mary to the local clinic where her leg ulcer would be dressed.

The leg ulcer dressing

If sufficient space is made to carry out the dressing, then the postural issues for staff are reduced immediately. The management of her pain, both from arthritis and the leg ulcer, will assist in Mary being able to move more comfortably for the staff.

The use of equipment such as the Community Nurse Leg Ulcer Kit can significantly reduce the strain on the nurse's back. This could be used in conjunction with some of the other kneeling systems such as the Ergokneeler described in Chapter 60. The ability of the nurse to be able to change their posture when carrying out the dressing will reduce the risk of cumulative back injury.

The pressure on the nurse's knees throughout the procedure has to be addressed and even if there are no specific kneeling systems available the use of knee pads as shown in Chapter 60 can be a good risk-reducing measure.

The patient's mobility

Anything which helps maximise Mary's mobility will be helpful not only to the nurses, but to promote healing for Mary. In addition this may increase the quality of her life. The use of community physiotherapy and occupational therapy services can have a significant impact on the patient's quality of life and the ability to keep them in their own home.

Staff health

Staff need to be reminded of the problems of cumulative injury due to poor posture when carrying out techniques such as leg ulcer dressings in patients' homes. The ability to rotate staff round the more challenging dressing can be a simple way of

Moving and Handling Patients at a Glance. First Edition. Hamish MacGregor. © 2016 John Wiley & Sons, Ltd. Published 2016 by John Wiley & Sons, Ltd.

reducing risk. Having two people to carry out the task in some instances can sometimes be quicker and therefore reduces the strain for both the nurse and the patient.

Working in people's homes in general
There are often negotiations and compromises to be made when working in people's homes. In the scenario above this is the patient's home, but it is the nurses' place of work. It is for this reason moving and handling risk assessments need to be carried out and regularly reviewed. This will ensure that high risk activities are not accepted, while the patient's dignity and right to choice is acknowledged.

Table CS2 The component parts in a moving and handling risk assessment (see Chapter 7 for more details)

The Task

Factors that may need to be considered	Risk-reducing measures	Equipment issues
• Can you apply the key safe principles of handling? (see Chapter 5)	Ensure staff are trained, competent and posturally aware	
• Be aware of static postures (see Chapter 4)	Ensure staff are trained, competent and posturally aware	
• Can you avoid twisting?	Ensure staff are trained, competent and posturally aware	
• Do you need to carry over a long distance?	Moving the bucket of water on a trolley rather than carrying it	
• Are there unpredictable movement of loads?	Not applicable	
• Does this involve repetitive handling?	Rotate staff round the leg ulcer dressings that are more problematic	
• Are there sufficient breaks factored into the task?	Ensure breaks are taken at regular intervals	

Individual capability

Factors that may need to be considered	Risk-reducing measures	Equipment issues
• Require a certain level of fitness?	Are staff encouraged to keep themselves fit?	
• Present a risk to those who have pre-existing health problems?	Ensure that no staff with a current or pre-existing musculoskeletal problem works with the patient on a regular basis. Staff with knee problems as well as back problems can be more at risk	Suitable kneeling equipment is available; see Chapter 60 for more detail
• Constitute a hazard to those who are pregnant?	Pregnant staff should have had a pregnancy risk assessment. See HSE flow chart: www.hse.gov.uk/mothers/docs/pregnant-workers-flow-chart.pdf	
• Require specialised training?	Additional training may be required for some staff and a review of other options available to make this safer	Additional training on the use of equipment may be required
• Require a certain level of knowledge, skills and competency?	Ensure staff are trained, competent and posturally aware	
• Become more risky at certain times of the day?	N/A	

The load

Factors that may need to be considered	Risk-reducing measures	Equipment issues
• Heavy?	Moving a bucket of water on a trolley rather than carrying it	Having a trolley available
		Hose to attach to the tap
	Having a hose to connect to the tap in order to eliminate the need to lift a bucket in and out of the bath	Having a back pack on wheels available
	Carrying equipment in a back pack with wheels may make the transporting of equipment into the patient's home safer	
	Also see person section below	
• Bulky?		
• Difficult to grasp?		
• Unstable or have an uneven weight distribution?		
• Potentially harmful, for example, hot		

Person factors

Factors that may need to be considered	Risk-reducing measures	Equipment issues
• The patient's leg is having to be moved which can be heavy and bulky	Ensure the patient is in the best position to carry out the procedure	See equipment section below
• Medical conditions that will affect handling	The addressing of Mary's mobility issue is important. An Occupational Therapy assessment to review Aids to Daily Living may be needed. A community physiotherapy assessment to improve mobility	
• Level of understanding?	Not applicable	
• Level of cooperation?	See pain control below	
• Conscious level	Not applicable	
• Pain	Adequate pain control must be given before the dressing is carried out as this may increase Mary's ability to cooperate	
• Attachments, i/v lines, catheters, drains	Not applicable	

The environment

Factors that may need to be considered	Risk-reducing measures	Equipment issues
• Is there enough space?	Obtaining agreement to remove some clutter from the room	
• Type of flooring?	Obtaining agreement to remove loose rugs from the floor	
• Are there stairs to be negotiated?	Not applicable	
• Is there a good ergonomic layout?	Look at all activities to be carried out and see if there are further things that can be moved from the area	
• Are there obstacles in the way?	Remove as necessary before any move is carried out	
• Is the temperature conducive to the work being carried out?	As Mary likes to keep the house warm due her immobility staff to keep themselves well hydrated	
• Is there sufficient lighting?	Ensure there is good lighting	

Equipment

Factors that may need to be considered	Risk-reducing measures	Equipment issues
• Is it appropriate for the task?	Ensure all necessary equipment is sourced	The use of a system such as the Community Nurse Leg Ulcer Kit from Carbonlite Medical. See link below www.youtube.com/watch?v=6cAz7RE7Eco Other kneeling solution (see Chapter 60)
• Has the safe working load been identified?	If using a system to hold the patient's leg ensure it can take the weight of the patient's leg	
• Is it in good working order and free from damage?	Staff made aware of need to check equipment before it is used	
• Has it been serviced/checked in accordance with legal requirements, for example, LOLER? (see Chapter 2)	Not applicable	
• Do the staff require any special training to operate the equipment?	Additional training on equipment may be required	

Other influencing factors

Factors that may need to be considered	Risk-reducing measures	Equipment issues
• Levels of stress or other psychosocial factors	Are there policies in place to manage staff who may be experiencing stress?	
• Poor staffing levels supplemented by high numbers of agency staff	If this is an ongoing issue are there robust systems in place to record, monitor and escalate staffing problems to senior management	
• Pressures of work or at home	Staff feel comfortable to discuss these issues with manager	
• Organisational policies	Ensure there is appropriate policy and protocols for the management of leg ulcers in the community	

Index

Moving and Handling Patients at a Glance. First Edition. Hamish MacGregor. © 2016 John Wiley & Sons, Ltd. Published 2016 by John Wiley & Sons, Ltd.